Medical Aspects of

Beekeeping

Other books by Harry Riches

Bee Keeping W. & G. Foyle Ltd, London 1976

Honey Marketing Bee Books New & Old, Burrowbridge, Somerset
1989

A Handbook of Beekeeping Northern Bee Books, Hebden Bridge
1992

Mead - Making, Exhibiting and Judging Bee Books New & Old,
Charlestown, Cornwall 1997

Medical Aspects of

Beekeeping

Harry R. C. Riches, MD FRCP

Northern Bee Books

Published by Northern Bee Books
Scout Bottom Farm
Mytholmroyd
Hebden Bridge, HX7 5JS

ISBN 0-907908-94-2

Printed by LightningSource

CONTENTS

Acknowledgments.

I am grateful to John Kinross of Bee Books New & Old for encouraging me to write this small book and for other help and advice he gave me.

I also appreciate the kindness of the Editors of *Bee World* and *Bee Craft* for allowing me to reproduce material I originally published in their journals.

My thanks are due to my daughter Penelope for her help in correcting the draft manuscript and for proof-reading.

Finally, I must also thank all those beekeepers who, with great patience, courtesy and fortitude, have listened to my talks on allergy problems associated with our craft. Optimistically, my hope is that the deficiencies of my past lectures will be remedied by the current publication.

H.R.

Preface

Over the years I have written a number of articles on medical problems associated with insect stings. These were published in both medical and beekeeping journals, but with the passage of time some are no longer easily available. However, I still get a small steady flow of requests for information and it is this which nurtured the idea that I should put together a collection of my main publications. This small book is an attempt to fulfill that objective.

I have had a life-long interest in bees. It started as a boy when I used to watch with fascination my grandfather manipulating his skeps of bees. We lived in a village in Norfolk and I recall that he sold his honey in the 1930's for 1/3d per pound i.e. equivalent to 6p in the current funny money! I still remember with pride my first solo hiving of a swarm over fifty years ago.

My beekeeping activities (but not my interest) had to be curtailed when I began my medical career but even then beekeeping occasionally came into the picture, sometimes to my advantage! One such piece of luck occurred in 1942. Guy's Hospital Medical School, where I was a student, was evacuated to Tunbridge Wells during the War. One of the professors, a delightful man, took up beekeeping and because he was a novice I was able to help. I became his blue-eyed boy which possibly eased my passage through Guy's!

Another incident imprinted in my memory occurred when I was a House Physician at the Brompton Hospital in 1952. A male patient was admitted to my ward suffering from advanced ankylosing spondylitis, a disease causing solid rigidity of the spine. Its cause is unknown but many consider it a form of rheumatoid arthritis of the spine. The poor man had had every type of treatment which was

1

available and, in addition, stated to my great surprise that he had also had bee sting therapy. I was enthralled and asked where. He said a practitioner in Notting Hill Gate treated him three times each week. I was amazed when he told me that he paid 2 guineas each session, i.e. £6-6-0 per week. He was a manual worker probably earning £6 to £8 per week and admitted that nearly all his wages went to pay for the treatment. In a jocular vein I said to him - if you want bee sting therapy why not find a beekeeper he would let you stick your backside into the front of a hive for nothing! (This may sound vulgar but is anatomically appropriate positioning because ankylosing spondylitis usually starts in the joints at the bottom of the spine!!) He looked at me as if I was completely ignorant about bees and explained that the bees the practitioner used were "special medicated bees". I fear he was stung in more ways than one! I have to confess that this early experience has left me with a degree of scepticism about bee sting therapy since it did not help that poor man in the slightest and I found it repugnant that an impecunious and seriously disabled person was relieved of so much money.

A seminal period occurred in my beekeeping activities about thirty years ago when I became allergic to stings. It first manifested itself as gross local swelling. For example, if I was stung on the ankle my leg became so swollen by the following day that it would be difficult to put on my trousers. The culmination came when after a single sting on a finger whilst manipulating a colony in my garden I collapsed unconscious. I remember slowly recovering looking up to find my two small children peering down at me convulsed in laughter shouting "get a doctor", then to peels of laughter saying "he is a doctor"! To them the thought of getting a doctor to a doctor seemed very comical! I recovered in a few minutes but the experience made me realize that I must do something about my venom sensitivity. Following the orthodox medical view that it is not a good idea to treat oneself, I wrote to a very distinguished allergist at the Brompton Hospital under whom I had trained. I recall vividly reading his reply the gist of which was "Harry, you should give up beekeeping". I think my wife was taken aback when I tore up the letter in rage muttering "the silly ------ doesn't know anything about it"!

Allergy training at the Brompton Hospital was very much focussed on diseases such as asthma and other more exotic allergic lung disorders. I decided, therefore, that I had to find out myself about insect venom sensitivity by reading all the available literature, after which I would treat myself. There was no way that I was going to give up my bees.

At that time Whole Body Extract of bees was in use for purposes of hyposensitization treatment. It was given by injection in gradually increasing dosage. I decided to give myself a course but modified the standard recommended procedure by taking an anti-histamine tablet an hour before giving myself the injections. My reason for doing this was based on the well known fact that histamine release is a fundamental feature in anaphylaxis so it seemed worthwhile to block its effects by use of an anti-histamine.

I completed the course with no problems but during the next beekeeping season I always took an anti-histamine tablet before attending my hives. I had no serious reactions from stings and subsequently stopped taking the tablets. For more than twenty five years I have had no recurrence of venom sensitivity.

Looking back it is interesting to note that it was later shown that Whole Body Extract of bees is ineffective in treating venom sensitivity. Subsequently, another cogent finding was that in animal experiments anti-histamines had a considerable protective effect when given **prior** to challenge with an allergen to which the experimental animals had been sensitized. The question, therefore, which remains in my mind is, did I become immune to stings as a natural phenomenon, or did I desensitize myself to venom whilst under the protective benefit of anti-histamines? I will never know.

I suppose it reasonable to ask why I have described the above events at such length. My hope is that it will convince the reader that I am a beekeeper of some seniority and that advice I give about allergy problems is based on medical knowledge together with personal experience of venom hypersensitivity and anaphylaxis. I include details of the man with ankylosing spondylitis so that the reader may be aware of the unfortunate experience which has undoubtedly fostered my cautious approach to bee sting therapy and may. well have left me with a degree of prejudice against the treatment.

Harry Riches
Northwood
October 2000

Chapter 1.

Stings

At best, stings are nothing more than a trivial hurt: at worst, in rare circumstances, they cause serious illness and may prove fatal. Sadly, there are on average four or five deaths each year in the U.K. attributed to insect stings. These dramatic incidents attract wide publicity in the news media and consequently cause considerable concern and apprehension, especially to those members of the general public who have a limited knowledge of bees and wasps. Some lurid reports in the media have been grossly inaccurate. For example, a few years ago a national newspaper featured a story about an elderly lady who was alleged to have died after being attacked by a swarm of bees whilst she was on her way to a wedding. The truth was quite different! A Coroners Inquest established that the lady had died from natural causes and there was no evidence that she had been stung! It was a matter of conjecture that fear when she saw the swarm had precipitated a heart attack. Although the inaccuracy of the original report was brought to the attention of the newspaper, the editor declined to publish a correction. Presumably there is no sales benefit in correcting yesterday's errors!

If for no better reason than self protection, it is highly desirable that beekeepers have some knowledge of the effects of stings and their possible dangers. Self interest should not, however, be the only consideration. Beekeepers can, and should, use their unique position and knowledge to educate the general public about bees and help to allay exaggerated fears and superstitions.

It is very difficult to determine the true incidence of stings in the general population because the majority of those afflicted are likely to treat themselves with home remedies. Only serious reactions come to the attention of a doctor. However, a survey was commissioned by a pharmaceutical company in Great Britain in 1981 for market research purposes in which 3000 individuals were interviewed. The findings suggested that about 10% of the population are stung each year by bees or wasps and that some 40,000 suffer reactions of sufficient severity to merit further investigation. Surveys in some other parts of the world have suggested that serious reactions to stings are more frequent. In U.S.A. medical circles, for example, it is widely accepted that between 1% and 2% of the population may be at risk. Whatever the true figure it is clear that a significant number of individuals suffer unpleasant reactions when stung.

Before considering the reactions caused by stings it is desirable to have some basic knowledge of the sting organ and the composition of bee venom.

The Sting Organ.

In evolutionary history the sting apparatus of the honey bee (Apis mellifera) evolved from an ovipositor. The latter was used by primitive bees to deposit eggs in crevices or other protective places. However, when Apis mellifera developed the social habit of living in a colony and rearing brood in combs, an ovipositor was no longer a general requirement. The ability to defend the nest, however, became essential and in the course of time the redundant ovipositor in the worker caste evolved into a defensive weapon, the sting apparatus The evolution of the sting from the ovipositor of the female egg laying caste explains the absence of a sting in the male drone.

The sting organ of the bee is complex. Those requiring a detailed description are referred to books on bee anatomy. The following is a very simplified basic description.

The sting of the honey bee is contained within a chamber at the end of the abdomen from which it can be protruded. For purposes of description it can be divided into two main parts: one is the basal part which is the principal motor apparatus containing the muscles for protruding and thrusting the sting into an enemy, together with glands which produce venom and alarm pheremones: the other part is the tapering shaft, about 2 mm long, which is the piercing instrument. The structure of the latter is interesting and functionally important. The shaft consists of a sheaf of three components which together taper to a sharp point. The upper single component is the stylet and below are two barbed lancets. In the centre of the shaft between these components is the channel through which venom passes. The slender lancets are held close to the undersurface of the stylet in groves. When activated, the lancets slide back and forth alternately and because of the backward direction of their barbs, which prevent retraction, they tend to be propelled further into the victim. Remarkably, the bee is able to withdraw its sting from insect enemies but not from man and other mammals with elastic skins. In its struggle to withdraw its sting from a mammal the entire sting apparatus is frequently torn from the bee, a mortal injury, but the penetrating movements of the lancets continue for up to a minute driving them further into the victim and increasing envenomation. At the same time as the sting organ is injecting venom it liberates alarm pheremones into the atmosphere. These are attractants, which in effect recruit other bees to attack. Clearly, therefore, a beekeeper is well advised to manipulate colonies carefully and use smoke judiciously so as to minimize disturbance in the knowledge that one sting is likely to provoke many more.

Venom

Venom glands begin to function soon after an adult bee emerges, with maximum production being achieved in a further two to three weeks. The venom sac of a fully mature worker bee will contain between 100 and 150 microgrammes of venom of which approximately 50 microgrammes is injected in a sting.

Bee venom is a complex mixture of pharmacologically and biochemically active proteins and peptides, together with a number of smaller molecular substances. Since it is largely water (88%) it follows that the solid components, which are present in small quantity, are extremely potent.

The main solid constituents are the enzymes Phospholipase A, Hyaluronidase, and Acid Phosphatase, together with the toxic peptides Melittin, Apamin, Mast Cell Degranulating Peptide, Secapin, and Tertiapin. The small molecular substances found in trace amounts include Histamine, Dopamine and Noradrenaline.

Phospholipase A destroys phospholipids which are essential components of cell membranes. There are numerous phospholipases in the animal kingdom; that found in bee venom is one of the most potent.

Hyaluronidase breaks down hyaluronic acid which is the interstitial ground substance of tissues which binds cells together. This destructive action allows injected venom to spread easily and quickly from its point of entry. It can be conveniently described as a 'spreading agent.'

Acid Phosphatase splits phosphate from organic compounds.

Melittin has a destructive action on many body cells including blood cells, its potency being enhanced by the presence of Phospholipase A.

Apamin is toxic to the nervous system with effects similar to a potent snake venom neurotoxin.

Mast Cell degranulating peptide (MCD peptide) is capable of liberating histamine from Mast Cells. The latter are found throughout the body but are particularly concentrated in airways, blood vessels, gut and skin. When liberated, histamine causes profound changes in those organs, notably constriction of airways and dilatation of blood vessels.

Other peptides (Secapin, Tertiapin etc.) are present in small amounts and appear to have only a low toxicity to mammals.

The small molecular substances present in trace quantity are vaso-active amines. Their importance has not been clearly defined but it seems likely that they act as adjuvants to the major toxins in venom.

The effects of stings

The small quantity of venom injected in a single sting is sufficient to kill or immobilize insect enemies of similar size to the bee. As far as man is concerned, however, with a huge body mass compared with the bee, a single sting is but a minor painful experience. However, serious toxic effects may occur if perchance multiple stings are sustained in a brief period of time, so that mass envenomation occurs. In such circumstances fatalities are possible from the direct poisonous effects of venom. It has been calculated that the Median Lethal Dose (L.D.50) of bee venom for an average sized adult is between 500 and

1000 stings. Although some have survived many more, the sensible and obvious conclusion is that multiple stings must be avoided.

The reaction to a sting in a <u>normal non-allergic and non-immune individual</u> shows a typical sequence of changes.

1. First, there is pain at the site of entry. (*The embedded sting should be brushed out as quickly as possible*)

2. Within a minute or so a raised white bleb will appear, often 1 to 2 cms in diameter.

3. Soon after, an area of perhaps 5 to 10 cms in diameter surrounding the raised bleb will become red and hot with moderate swelling.

4. It may take 24 to 48 hours for all the swelling to disappear.

The amount of swelling caused by a sting in a normal non-allergic, non-immune individual is strongly influenced by the toughness and laxity of the skin where it enters. For example, on the sole of the foot where the skin is tough, a sting will be painful but swelling will be very little. On the other hand, stings in the soft skin of the face and neck will cause considerable swelling.

The response to a sting in an allergic individual may be quite violently different from the above and will be described in a subsequent chapter. In contrast, a person, such as an experienced beekeeper, who has developed immunity may show very little reaction when stung. This also will be explained later.

Certain critical sites, such as the inside of the mouth and throat, are very dangerous places to be stung because of the massive swelling o very soft tissues which may ensue. This could be fatal if of sufficient extent to block the airway.

Another critical site is the eyeball. If a sting penetrates into the eyeball the injected venom could induce a very fierce inflammatory reaction within the eye, sufficient to permanently damage sight.

For these two important reasons I take the view that beekeepers should always wear a veil when manipulating bees.

Treatment

The important essential first treatment of a bee sting is to remove the embedded sting as quickly as possible. This is easily done by scraping it out with the finger nail or by simply brushing it off with the hand. Do not delay by looking for tweezers in order to grasp the sting. Although it is arguable whether grasping a sting will cause more venom to be injected there is no doubt that delay in removal is highly detrimental.

All sorts of remedies have been advised as beneficial applications to relieve the pain and swelling of stings, usually based on anecdotal evidence. These include honey, propolis extract, blue bag, mallow leaves and other herbal products, meat tenderiser, antihistamine cream etc.,etc.. As far as I am aware, these have not been subjected to critical scientific appraisal so it is difficult to know whether they do any good. A note of caution is necessary about the use of antihistamine creams. The occasional use of such products does not normally cause problems but if used repeatedly they can themselves cause a severe skin sensitivity rash (contact dermatitis) in a minority of individuals. The trouble caused could be worse than the sting! For that reason most dermatologists do not favour the application of antihistamine products to the skin.

Normally, no special local applications are required but something soothing such as a cold compress, or calamine lotion will help. A couple of aspirin tablets by mouth will lessen discomfort and inflammation. If swelling is extensive, hot, and itchy, a steroid cream application such as Betnovate is useful.

Facts to remember

♦ Insect stings are common

♦ Four or five deaths occur annually on average in U.K. from insect stings.

♦ Bee venom is a complex mixture of enzymes and toxic proteins.

♦ Stings are especially dangerous in the mouth and eyeball.

♦ A veil should always be worn when opening a hive.

The following chapter is essentially a reprint of my article which appeared in Bee World, a journal of the International Bee Research Association,18 North Road,Cardiff,CF1 3DY,UK

Chapter 2.

Hypersensitivity To Bee Venom

A feature of medical progress in recent years has been an impressive increase in knowledge of immunological mechanisms and their role in the pathogenesis of disease. Studies of hypersensitivity to insect venoms have contributed to the understanding of these mechanisms and have also demonstrated effective methods for protecting people who suffer unpleasant symptoms when stung. Most of this research has been published in specialist medical and scientific journals, and for that reason is not easily available to the general reader. The purpose of the present review, therefore, is to outline the important advances which are likely to be helpful to beekeepers, especially those who are apprehensive about the risks and complications of stings.

The concepts of allergy and anaphylaxis were formulated at the beginning of 20th century. In 1902 Charles Richet, a French pathologist, tried to make a dog immune to jellyfish poison by giving it small sublethal doses. The idea was not original: in fact, it was 2000 years old and derived from the experiments of a notorious Persian, Mithridates, King of Pontus in Asia Minor. This unpleasant man was intensely interested in poisons and accrued much knowledge by experimenting on his prisoners of war. He established that by repeatedly administering small doses of poison, tolerance could be achieved so that eventually a known lethal dose could be taken without serious consequences. Copying this procedure, Richet gave a dog a sublethal dose of jellyfish poison by injection and 22 days

13

later repeated the dose. The death of the animal immediately after the second theoretically sublethal injection confounded him because the dog had clearly become more susceptible to the poison, and not tolerant. After further experiments he concluded that whereas a moderately toxic substance when *first* injected may only produce minor symptoms, serious illnes and even death may result if a *second* similar injection is given after an interval of time. For this phenomenon Richet proposed the term anaphylaxis. Soon after these observations relating to toxic substances were accepted, Maurice Arthus, another French physiologist, made the important discovery in 1903 that anaphylaxis could also be triggered by non-toxic protein products such as horse serum and cow's milk.

At about the same time von Pirquet, an Austrian paediatrician, noted that some diphtheria patients, after receiving anti-toxin, developed fever, swollen glands and skin rashes. Investigation led him to conclude that these reactions were caused by the horse serum in the preparation and not the anti-toxin component. To designate this altered reaction von Pirquet coined the word allergy. As originally defined the term allergy includes both *decreased* altered capacity to react (e.g. the failure to react to diphtheria toxin in subjects with antibodies against it) and *increased* capacity to react (e.g. in subjects with hypersensitivity responses to environmental allergens etc.). By common usage the response in which there is decreased altered capacity to react is described as *immunity*, whilst increased altered capacity to react is designated *hypersensitivity or allergy*. In this context the terms allergy and hypersensitivity are used synonymously.

It is well known that patients who have recovered from an infectious disease such as measles seldom suffer a second attack. The immunity achieved is specific to that particular disease being dependent upon protective antibodies which Tiselius and Kabat demonstrated were present in the gamma globulin fraction of serum proteins. Gamma globulin antibodies are usually referred to as immunoglobulins. In man, five major structural types or classes of immunoglobulins have been distinguished, namely immunoglobulin A (abbreviated to IgA),

14

immunoglobulin D (IgD), immunoglobulin E (IgE), immunoglobulin G (IgG) and immunoglobulin M (IgM). IgG accounts for approximately 80% of the total immunoglobulin in the serum of a normal adult and is itself divided into four sub-classes with differences in chemical structure and biological behaviour. The other immunoglobulins are present in approximately the following proportions: IgA 13%, IgM 6%, IgD 1%, and only traces of IgE.

Each class of immunoglobulin has its own particular function. In response to bacterial invasion IgM and IgG antibodies are synthesized and circulate freely in the blood and tissue fluids. IgA provides defence against invasion by micro-organisms at body surfaces, and is notably present in saliva, tears, sweat, and in the secretions of the respiratory and alimentary tracts. The function of IgD is not clearly known. Only a very small quantity of IgE is present in the blood of a normal adult, but a considerable increase has been observed in those suffering from parasitic infestation, especially intestinal worms. Because of this it has been postulated that IgE may have a defensive role against parasitic diseases. Although IgE is produced in excess in those with certain allergic disorders, it is not easily detected in the blood because it does not circulate freely in the body fluids but attaches itself to special receptor sites on the surface of basophil leucocytes of the blood, and on mast cells which are widely distributed in the skin, respiratory tract and gut. This unique arrangement has great physiological importance which in simplified terms can be described as follows.

Individuals who suffer from certain allergic disorders such as hay fever, pollen asthma, food and drug allergies, sting allergy, etc have a genetic predisposition to produce IgE antibodies in excess when exposed to certain substances which are 'foreign' to their bodies. For example, on initial exposure to grass pollen a person destined to suffer from hay fever will generate IgE anti-bodies specific to grass pollen which will attach to their mast cells and basophils. These attached anti-bodies will also lock on to pollen should it come into proximity at a later date. The combination of IgE and pollen occurring at the surface of a mast cell has a damaging effect on its cell wall. This triggers enzyme systems within the cell resulting in the liberation into the circulation of pharmacologically active substances such as histamine, serotonin, slow reacting substance of anaphylaxis and prostaglandins. These very potent vasoactive agents are responsible for the general and local manifestations of an acute allergic reaction.

The following are diagrammatic illustrations of the interaction of IgE and IgG anti-bodies, venom and mast cells

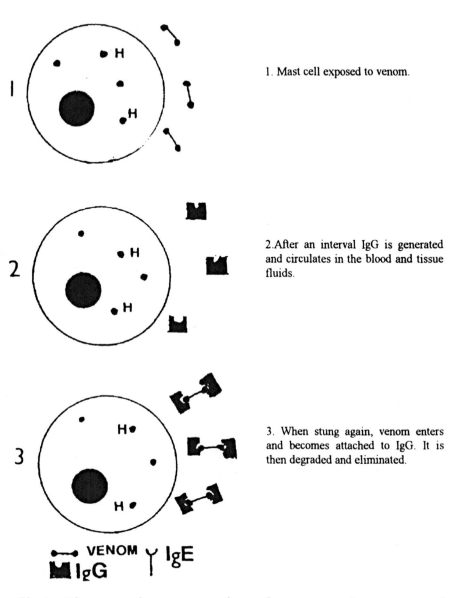

1. Mast cell exposed to venom.

2. After an interval IgG is generated and circulates in the blood and tissue fluids.

3. When stung again, venom enters and becomes attached to IgG. It is then degraded and eliminated.

●━━● VENOM   Υ IgE
◼ IgG

Fig.1. Diagrammatic representation of a mast cell, venom and antibodies in a subject who develops immunity.

17

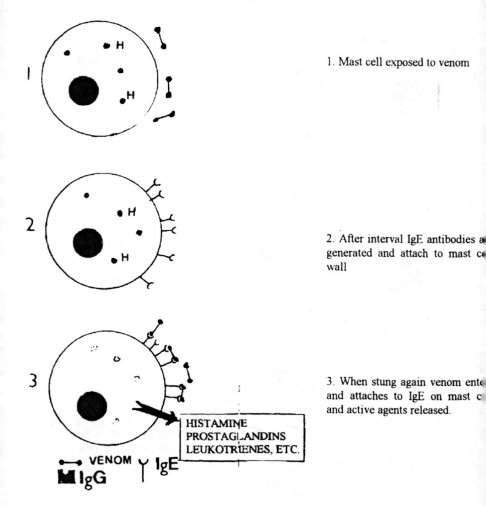

1. Mast cell exposed to venom

2. After interval IgE antibodies a
generated and attach to mast ce
wall

3. When stung again venom ente
and attaches to IgE on mast c
and active agents released.

HISTAMINE
PROSTAGLANDINS
LEUKOTRIENES, ETC.

VENOM Y IgE
IgG

Fig.2. Diagrammatic representation of a mast cell, venom, a
antibodies in a subject developing hypersensitivity.

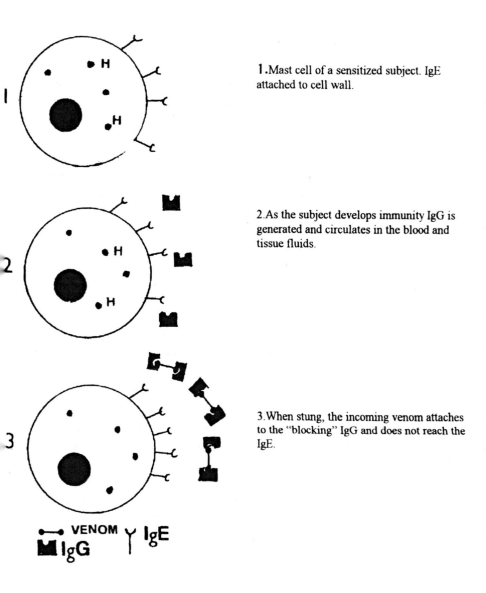

1. Mast cell of a sensitized subject. IgE attached to cell wall.

2. As the subject develops immunity IgG is generated and circulates in the blood and tissue fluids.

3. When stung, the incoming venom attaches to the "blocking" IgG and does not reach the IgE.

VENOM Y IgE
IgG

Fig.3. Diagrammatic representation of a mast cell, venom, and antibodies in an allergic subject developing immunity.

Immunoglobulin antibodies are synthesized by lymphocytes and plasma cells which are present in the blood and reticulo-endothelial system. In man there are two main categories of lymphocytes, designated T and B. The B series mature to become plasma cells and are entirely concerned with the production of humoral antibodies (immunoglobulins), whilst T lymphocytes (thymus dependent) are concerned with cell-mediated immunity, the activity which causes so much difficulty in the rejection of transplanted organs. T cells have an additional function in that they influence the activity of B cells; some have a 'helper' function and facilitate the production of antibodies, whilst others, described as 'suppressors', discourage the output of antibodies. Clearly, the balance of activity between 'helper' and 'suppressor' T cells has a critical influence on antibody production.

To evoke an immune response a substance has to possess certain essential qualities. A fundamental prerequisite for immunogenicity is that a substance must be 'foreign' to the recipient. The most potent immunogenic substances are proteins of high molecular weight: those with a molecular weight below 5000 seldom trigger reactions. Other factors which influence an immune response are the molecular rigidity and complexity of a substance, the method and route of administration, and the dose.

Having described the basic biochemical components of immune responses it is now appropriate to consider examples of reactions which occur in experimental animals when challenged with immunogenic agents.

Different animal species show wide variation in their immunological responses to antigenic substances as illustrated by the two following examples.

If a rabbit is given an injection of a bacterial toxoid, which is a 'foreign' protein substance to the rabbit, IgM antibodies will appear in its serum after a few days. A short time later IgG antibodies will also be detected. The response to this first injection (primary immunization) is delayed and quantitatively small. If a second dose of the same toxoid is given 3 or 4 weeks later the response will be much different. Following this injection (secondary immunization) there will be a prompt and much increased rise in antibodies which will be predominantly of the IgG type. If further injections are given at similar intervals the responses will be equally brisk and the rise in IgG antibodies considerable. Throughout this procedure the animal has not been harmed; it has in fact benefited because it has acquired resistance (immunity) to infection by the bacterium from which the toxoid was made.

An entirely different response is elicited from a guinea-pig when challenged with a foreign substance. If a healthy guinea-pig is given a small quantity of egg albumen (1mg) by injection, it will not show any visible ill effects. However, if a similar small dose of egg albumen is injected after an interval of three weeks the response will be dramatically different. Within minutes of the injection the animal will have difficulty breathing and may collapse and die quickly. The animal has, in fact, suffered a classical acute anaphylactic reaction. This catastrophic self-destruction occurred because the guinea-pig responded to the intrusion of egg albumen by generating IgE type antibodies rather than the protective IgG and IgM varieties.

Activation of the IgE system, as demonstrated in the above guinea-pig experiment, is the type of hypersensitivity which is involved in sting allergy of beekeepers. There are, however, other forms of allergic reactions which are dependent on different mechanisms.

Based on differences in pathogenesis, Gell and Coombs classified allergic reactions into **four** principal types.

A reactions which results from antigen interacting with IgE antibodies bound to mast cells, with consequent release of histamine and other pharmacolgically active substances as previously enumerated is described as **Type 1**. Anaphylaxis, as exemplified by the response of the guinea-pig to injections of egg albumen, as previously noted, is the most dramatic and extreme manifestation of this type of hypersensitivity. Less severe IgE-mediated reactions in humans include general symptoms such as faintness, nausea, vomiting, respiratory difficulty and skin rashes. Minor reactions are swelling and erythema (redness) at the site of contact with the antigen.

Type 2 and **Type 4** reactions will not be considered further because insect venom does not appear to provoke them.

Type 3 reactions must be considered because they are the basis of some delayed complications of stings. They occur when antigen combines with a specific circulating antibody of the IgG class known as a precipitin. This results in antigen/antibody aggregates in the circulation and tissues, with activation of the complement system leading to the liberation of tissue-damaging enzymes and other mediators of inflammation. In simple terms, the complement system is a series of interacting proteins which are normally found in the circulation in inactive form. When activated, a number of biological consequences ensue including damage to cell walls causing cell death. This attracts polymorphonuclear leucocytes, the classical cells of inflammation, and at the same time chemical agents of inflammation, such as prostaglandins, are released.

Clinically, Type 3 reactions take two forms. If there is an excess of circulating precipitating antibodies, an injection of antigen will result in an erythematous (red) and oedematous (swollen) local reaction which reaches its maximum in 3 to 8 hours, and may take many hours to resolve. This is known as the Arthus reaction. Histologically the lesion is characterized by an intense infiltration with inflammatory cells, mainly polymorphonuclear leucocytes. The alternative variety of Type 3 reaction occurs if there is a great excess of antigen present as happens when a

22

large dose of 'foreign' protein is injected. An illness, described as serum sickness may develop some 7 to 10 days after the injection, manifested by swollen lymph glands, skin rashes, and joint pains. The illness may persist many days.

Having described the essential mechanisms of immunological responses in general terms, it is now appropriate to relate that information to reactions which bee venom may evoke in man. Bee venom has all the prerequisites of a potent allergen in that it is a 'foreign' substance consisting of a complex mixture of toxic proteins and peptides, many of high molecular weight, and possessing a wide variety of pharmacological properties.

Constituents of honeybee venom so far identified are three enzymes phospholipase A, hyaluronidase and acid phosphatase, together with the toxic proteins and peptides allergen C, melittin, melittin-F, apamin, mast cell degranulating peptide, secapin, tertiapin and traces of small molecular substances including histamine, dopamine and noradrenaline. Of these various components it appears that hyaluronidase, phospholipase A, acid phosphatase, allergen C and melittin are the main allergens.

Clinical Presentation of bee venom hypersensitivity

Type 1 Reactions
It is convenient to describe three types of manifestation of IgE-mediated bee venom hypersensitivity, namely, (a) large local reactions, (b) systemic reactions, and (c) anaphylaxis.   Such a classification is useful for purposes of description but it must be emphasized that the various reactions indicated are nothing more than differing degrees of severity of the same immunological process and not distinct unrelated disorders. Unfortunately, a progressive increase of severity of reactions is shown by some individuals during the course of a single beekeeping season. Their initial response to stings may be unremarkable but subsequent stings

provoke more swelling and with further exposure general symptoms occur and ultimately anaphylaxis. Fortunately, this sequence of events is not common.

It has been suggested that, in some circumstances, the quantity of venom injected and the site of entry may influence the severity of an ensuing reaction. In this context, stings on the face or neck seem prone to evoke serious reactions, a feature which may be related to the high blood supply of that area and the high concentration of mast cells in the skin of those parts of the body.

(a) Large local reactions

Extensive local swelling associated with hypersensitivity occurs in two phases. The initial acute response appears immediately after a sting and presents as a white weal around the point of entry surrounded by a zone of redness and swelling which, after the elapse of a few minutes, may cover an area of several square centimetres.

The second phase begins three or four hours later with the appearance of far more extensive swelling. An affected part becomes red, itchy and tender. Swelling may take 12 hours to reach its maximum and two or three days to resolve. This secondary swelling is sometimes described as a 'late cutaneous reaction' and, like the initial response is IgE dependent. Whereas histamine release is predominantly responsible for the immediate reaction, it appears that other mediators which are slow-acting cause the delayed changes.

On most parts of the body swelling induced by stings is little more than a nuisance. However, in certain sites it can be dangerous. For example, a sting inside the mouth or throat may cause the soft tissues in those areas to swell so quickly and enormously that there is danger of respiratory obstruction.

As mentioned earlier, progressively increasing local reactions following stings are a matter of some concern because they may herald future systemic complications or anaphylaxis.

(b) Systemic reactions.

A general reaction typically occurs within a few minutes following a sting. The mildest symptoms are a general flushing of the skin, followed by an itchy nettle-rash (urticaria). More serious symptoms are chest wheeze (bronchospasm), nausea, vomiting, abdominal pains, palpitations and faintness. The speed of onset of these symptoms after a sting is a crude indicator of the likely severity of the problem; reactions occurring within a minute or two are likely to be serious, whilst delayed onset usually indicates a less serious outcome.

(c) Anaphylaxis

Anaphylaxis occurs within seconds or minutes of a sting. Since it may jeopardize life it must be considered a medical emergency. Common initial symptoms are chest wheeze, nausea, vomiting, confusion, followed by falling blood pressure which leads to unconsciousness. Death may result from circulatory collapse and respiratory obstruction.

In England and Wales official statistics indicate that insect stings are responsible, on average, for four or five deaths annually. In the U.S.A. between forty and fifty fatalities are attributed to this cause every year. Undoubtedly, anaphylaxis is responsible for most of these deaths.

Type 111 Reactions

(a) Arthus type
Typically, this reaction causes swelling which slowly develops to become apparent some eight to twelve hours after a sting, and may persist a few days. Bruising and blistering may occur in the immediate vicinity of the sting. Sometimes an indurated nodule or a sterile pustule may form where the sting entered and persist for several days. The classical Arthus reaction is caused by an excess of precipitins of the IgG class in the circulation combining with venom at the site of entry. It is difficult to differentiate this response from the late cutaneous reaction, previously described, which appears at roughly the same time after a sting, but has a different pathogenesis being IgE dependent. The occurrence of frank tissue damage such as bruising or blistering would suggest an Arthus reaction.

(b) Serum sickness type
This is not common and is perhaps more likely after an episode of multiple stings. Malaise, fever, joint pains, skin rashes, swelling of lymph nodes, and kidney disturbance (protein and blood in the urine), develop some three to ten days after stings and may persist several days.

(c) Other reactions
Very rarely, serious medical disorders such as encephalitis, polyneuritis, and renal failure have followed insect stings. These are usually thought to have a Type111 hypersensitivity pathogenesis. Although of medical importance and interest such complications are so rare that they will not be considered further here.

Natural History of bee venom allergy

Epidemiological studies of insect venom hypersensitivity in population groups in the U.S.A. have generally revealed a low incidence. Amongst 2010 Girl Scouts only 0.35% were sensitive to Hymenoptera stings and in a comparable group of 4992 Boy Scouts no more than 0.40% were afflicted. Similarly, of 3705 patients attending an allergy clinic in New England, only 0.38% gave a history of allergic symptoms related to Hymenoptera stings. In contrast with these low figures from North America, it has been reported that between 2% and 4% of the adult population in Switzerland have suffered allergic reactions following stings.

Although these findings are interesting, none of the studies indicate the number of individuals who had been stung. It therefore remains possible that the sensitivity of the majority of participants was never determined because they were not challenged. Recognizing that hypersensitivity is an immunological response which develops only after exposure to an allergen, studies which omit details of exposure are clearly open to criticism.

Because of their frequent exposure to stings, beekeepers are uniquely appropriate subjects in whom to study the natural history of insect venom hypersensitivity and immunity. The sequence of changes and the wide variation of responses to stings will be seen in any group of beginners during their first year or two in the craft. From the very outset some are fortunate and only experience tolerable pain and minimal swelling around the point of entry of a sting. Within a few months these lucky individuals can accept stings with composure. Their immunity is achieved by their ability to respond to the injected venom by generating predominantly IgG-type antibodies. Numerous studies have confirmed high levels of IgG and low levels of IgE in the blood of beekeepers who are immune to stings.

A second identifiable group amongst new beekeepers are those in whom the first few stings cause little disturbance, but with further exposure local swelling becomes a problem. The swellings may be unpleasant and unsightly, especially those on the face and neck. However, in the course of time reactions to stings gradually diminish and immunity is eventually achieved. This is the pattern of response in the majority of those starting beekeeping and it is gratifying that with a little stoicism the problem is usually overcome. Individuals who go through this pattern of response develop both IgE and IgG antibodies initially and slowly, over a varying period of time, and with repeated exposure to venom, the protective IgG antibodies become predominant with consequent relief of symptoms. Although IgE attached to mast cells and basophils persist in these individuals, any venom they encounter combines preferentially with their freely circulating IgG. In such circumstances IgG is often referred to as a 'blocking antibody', because it prevents, or blocks, the combination of venom with IgE.

The third group is a small minority who develop serious hypersensitivity to venom and may become dangerously ill if stung. In extreme circumstances death may ensue from acute anaphylaxis. Although this is an alarming possibility, some comfort can be derived from the knowledge that it is unusual for an individual to manifest serious hypersensitivity without some forewarning. Normally, those at risk show progressive worsening of their reactions to stings. Initially, local swelling may be extensive and each further sting produces more and more swelling until eventually, if exposure continues, general symptoms occur such as nausea, skin rash and respiratory difficulties. If these symptoms are ignored further stings may lead to collapse into unconsciousness, a classical feature of anaphylaxis, and a fatal outcome is then possible. Those who react badly to stings in this way do so because they develop large quantities of IgE antibodies and very little of the protective IgG type. It is interesting to speculate why this happens. Individuals with a personal history of hay fever, eczema, asthma, allergic rhinitis, and urticaria produce IgE in large quantities in response to a variety of environmental antigens. This constitutional tendency (described as atopy) is genetically controlled and genes associated with the disorder have been recognized. As a rough approximation, about 15% of the population have an atopic constitution and 50% of the children of two atopic parents will be similarly affected. Although the development of bee venom hypersensitivity is determined by genetic factors, not all those who suffer are atopic; in fact, in population groups studied, the incidence of Hymenoptera sting sensitivity was not apparently influenced by atopy. However, there is some evidence that if stings are repeatedly received, as by beekeepers and their families, those with an atopic constitution are more likely to develop hypersensitivity.

Diagnosis

History

In elucidating the cause of an allergic reaction, great importance is always attached to a careful history. The classical method is to formulate a strong clinical suspicion of the identity of the offending allergen from the history, and then confirm that it is responsible by special tests. Most people who are stung know whether the insect was a bee or a wasp, but some may not. Fortunately, for those who are hypersensitive investigation will determine the cause of the reaction, and will also provide a quantitative indication of the degree of sensitivity.

Skin tests

The simplest, cheapest, and most frequently used investigation in allergy diagnosis is the skin test. This, and the other tests used to confirm bee venom hypersensitivity, are dependent upon the presence of specific anti-bee venom IgE. To perform the test, a minute trace of dilute venom is introduced into the skin of the forearm, either by injection or by scratching or pricking through a droplet placed on the skin. All these techniques are effective, but in the U.K. the prick test is the most widely used. It gives few false positive results; is easily, cheaply, and painlessly performed; and there is little risk of provoking anaphylaxis in the test subject. For prick testing, pure venom in a dilution of $0.1\mu g/ml$ or $1\mu g/ml$ is used. Higher concentrations may give false positive results. The result is read within about 15 minutes of testing; a positive response is a weal surrounded by a red flare. The area of the weal gives a reasonably accurate indication of the degree of hypersensitivity. Sometimes, a few hours after the original reaction has resolved, a second swelling may appear that reaches its maximum in about 5 to 7 hours. This represents either a late cutaneous reaction or a Type 3 response.

Pure venom preparations are now used exclusively for skin testing, because purified specific allergens induce responses which are both sensitive and explicit, whereas substances of mixed composition, such as whole-body extracts of bees, give less reliable results. Absolute reliance should not, however, be placed on any single isolated skin test result because false positive and negative responses can occur. Skin test results should only be considered significant when corroborated by a good history or other investigations.

RAST test

The radioallergosorbent test (RAST) is a method for detecting specific IgE in blood. The principle of the test is that bee venom is coupled to an insoluble carrier and to it is added a drop of serum from the suspected allergic subject. If the serum contains anti-bee venom IgE, this will bind to the venom attached to the carrier. The presence of bound IgE is detected by its reaction with isotope-labelled antibody to IgE. After washing the carrier, the intensity of persisting radioactivity, determined by a gamma-ray counter, will be directly proportional to the quantity of specific IgE originally present in the serum sample.

The correlation between RAST tests and skin tests varies in different disorders. In bee venom hypersensitivity it is good; a typical study showed 91% correlation with 5% RAST positive only and 4% skin test positive only.

The RAST test has obvious disadvantages in that it requires a venous blood sample, it requires access to expensive laboratory equipment and technicians, and the result is not available for at least 24 hours. It has the advantage that it can be performed on those with skin disease or abnormality which makes skin testing inappropriate, and it also avoids exposing very highly sensitive individuals to tests with potentially hazardous allergens.

Histamine release from basophils

When washed leucocytes, including basophils, from an allergic subject are mixed with a dilute solution of the relevant allergen, histamine is released. This can be estimated fluorometrically. The test is specific for the allergen concerned and can be used to confirm bee venom hypersensitivity. Because the test requires technical laboratory facilities it has not become a routine clinical investigation, but remains a valuable research tool. Skin tests and histamine release studies using pure venom correlate well. Whole-body extracts of bees, however, fail to release histamine from basophils of subjects with bee sting sensitivity. Clearly, this is a strong indication that whole-body extracts of bees have no part to play in the treatment of venom allergy.

Treatment of bee venom allergy

It is convenient to consider treatment under three headings, namely
(a) immediate treatment following a sting
(b) prophylactic drug therapy
(c) immunotherapy

Immediate treatment following a sting

(i) *Local treatment*
A sting should be removed as quickly as possible by scraping it out with a finger nail or by brushing it out with the hand. The sting should not be grasped in an attempt to extract it as this causes delay and may squeeze more venom into the wound. After removal of the sting, calamine lotion or cold water compresses are effective soothing applications, but if the inflammation is severe a steroid cream can be applied. In addition to this local treatment aspirin by mouth (two 300mg tablets for an adult) would help to relieve pain and swelling providing, of course, the individual is not sensitive to aspirin!

Ointments, creams or sprays containing antihistamine preparations should not be used because their repeated application can cause severe skin sensitization. Dermatologists strongly deprecate the topical use of antihistamines for this reason.

A sting anywhere inside the mouth may cause such gross swelling of the soft tissues in that locality that respiratory obstruction can ensue and threaten life. Medical attention is therefore urgently required to maintain an airway. For an adult, a large dose of soluble steroid (e.g. methylprednisolone sodium succinate 125mg) should be given intravenously, together with an intramuscular injection of adrenaline 0.5mg to 1mg (0.5ml to 1.0ml of a 1 in 1000 solution). For children proportionately less is given according to age and weight.

The eye is another especially dangerous site for a sting. A sting in the eyeball is, fortunately, a rare event but when it happens it can cause such serious inflammation inside the eye that sight may be threatened. Furthermore, although only one eye may be directly injured by a sting, it is not uncommon for the other eye to react in similar fashion to the damaged one, a phenomenon known as sympathetic ophthalmitis.

Because of this risk to sight a veil should always be worn when manipulating bees.

(ii) *Treatment of systemic reactions*
The keystone of effective treatment of systemic reactions is adrenaline, the route of administration depending on the severity of symptoms. For those who suffer mild symptoms such as a minor chest wheeze, or an irritating skin rash, inhalation of an aerosol preparation of adrenaline acid tartrate (Medihaler-Epi, Riker Laboratories) should be adequate. When symptoms are more severe adrenaline should be given by injection subcutaneously, 0.5mg to 1mg as a 1 in 1000 solution for an adult, proportionately less for a child. An antihistamine such as Piriton (chlorpheniramine) 4mg by mouth, or 10mg by injection, is of little immediate benefit but helps to suppress skin rashes which may develop subsequently. Precharged syringes of adrenaline for self-administration are available on prescription, perhaps the best known in the U.K. is the 'EpiPen'. Beekeepers with significant hypersensitivity should consult their doctor with a view to obtaining a prescription and familiarize themselves with the technique of self-injection.

(iii) *Treatment of anaphylaxis*
Anaphylaxis is not common, but when it occurs it must be considered a major medical emergency which threatens life. Prompt and vigorous treatment is essential. Adrenaline 0.5mg to 1mg as a 1 in 1000 solution should be injected at once intramuscularly, followed by 10mg to 20mg of chlorpheniramine and 125mg of methylprednisolone sodium succinate intravenously. If there is no response to the above treatment in five minutes, or the patient deteriorates, the dose of adrenaline should be repeated. The victim should be placed in the recovery position, kept warm, clothing loosened, any dentures removed, and the airway kept clear. Such emergency treatment should be given at once, prior to transfer to hospital.

Prophylactic drug therapy

(i) *Antihistamines*
Although histamine is only one of the mediators of anaphylaxis it is probably the most important. Increased blood concentration of histamine during anaphylaxis have been described and appear to correlate well with the severity of symptoms. Antihistamines can, therefore, be expected to give some, but not complete, protection if taken *before* exposure to stings. Their absorption and distribution through the body are too slow for them to be of benefit in anaphylaxis if taken after being stung. For an adult, Piriton (chlorpheniramine) 4mg taken an hour or so before visiting the apiary would be suitable. A well known detrimental side effect of some antihistamines is drowsiness. It might, however, be argued that this property of mild sedation could benefit a sting sensitive beekeeper by helping to allay apprehension. The generally accepted prudent advice is that individuals should not drive motor vehicles under the influence of these drugs. (*See later article concerning newer non-sedating antihistamines.*)

(ii) *Mast-cell stabilizers*
Sodium cromoglycate (Intal) and ketotifen (Zaditen) are currently prescribed for the prevention of asthma attributable to inhaled allergens. Pharmacologically these drugs have a stabilizing effect on the cell membrane of mast cells, thereby preventing their degranulation and the subsequent release of histamine and other biologically active substance associated with IgE- mediated hypersensitivity reactions. However sodium cromoglycate has to be inhaled 3 or 4 times daily, and ketotifen must be taken twice daily orally for some weeks before a full therapeutic effect is achieved. Such treatment routines make these drug inappropriate for use in insect sting hypersensitivity.

Immunotherapy

(i)*Passively acquired immunity*

A susceptible individual who has been exposed to a common infectious diseases such as rubella (German measles) or hepatitis (infective jaundice) can be protected for a limited time against the development of those illnesses by injections of concentrated gamma globulin prepared from the blood of donors who have recovered from such diseases. This is now standard medical practice for certain risk categories.

Similarly, the blood of beekeepers who are immune to stings has been used experimentally to provide gamma globulin for the protection of those who are hypersensitive to bee venom. The therapeutic effectiveness of this gamma globulin is dependent upon its content of specific immunoglobulin G (IgG) Unfortunately, this passive transfer of antibodies from an immune individual to a vulnerable recipient provides only short-lived protection; at best a few weeks. It is unlikely to become a generally available treatment.

(ii) *Active hyposensitization*

Hyposensitization can be defined as the increase of clinical tolerance achieved in an allergic subject by the injection of increasing quantities of the specific allergen. In medical practice the technique was first used by Noon in 1911 for the prevention of hay fever. Much later, about thirty years ago, the treatment of insect sting allergy began, when whole-body extracts of bees and wasps became commercially available.

Although some allergists claimed satisfactory results using whole-body extracts, others questioned the potency of such preparations. Loveless and Fackler described the use of wasp venom in hyposensitization as long ago as 1956, but it was not until 1978 that the results of a properly controlled trial of immunotherapy using pure venom was published by Hunt and colleagues. This most important investigation showed conclusively that treatment with pure venom was effective in 95% cases, whereas whole-body extracts benefited only 36%; a percentage rather worse than the 42% who apparently improved with a placebo! Furthermore, the effectiveness of pure venom was confirmed by a significant rise in the blood level of IgG antibodies in those receiving venom, whilst those receiving whole-body extract or placebo showed no such change. The immunological incompetence of whole-body extracts as effective and relevant antigens in sting sensitivity has also been demonstrated by their failure to release histamine from venom-sensitized leucocytes in laboratory tests. Another important disadvantage of whole-body extracts is that they contain a multiplicity of insect proteins which are themselves capable of provoking additional allergy problems. In the light of mounting evidence of the effectiveness and safety of pure venoms, the Food and Drug Administration of the U.S.A. approved their clinical use in 1979 and in the following year they became available commercially in the U.K. Henceforth, only pure venoms should be used in skin tests and hyposensitization treatments for insect sting allergy. It is just possible that whole-body extracts may still find a limited use in the treatment of beekeepers who suffer symptoms akin to hay fever and asthma attributable to the inhalation of bee dust whilst manipulating colonies.

The selection of suitable candidates for immunotherapy is important. Obviously, those who suffer significant general symptoms should be treated. Extensive local swelling, however, is not an indication for immunotherapy despite it being so unpleasant that the victim may press for treatment. In this context it has to be remembered that the majority who suffer in this way will eventually develop immunity naturally.

My current advice to novice beekeepers who complain of extensive local swelling is to persevere, with the added precaution of taking an antihistamine tablet an hour before attending their apiary. This simple prophylactic treatment helps to limit swelling if stung and also gives some protection against a serious general reaction. In the course of time, when stings cause less swelling, the treatment can be withdrawn. There is no evidence that such prophylactic drug therapy suppresses or delays the development of natural immunity.

For those who suffer general symptoms, immunotherapy with pure venom is the treatment of choice. In this procedure, very small doses of venom are injected subcutaneously at regular intervals in gradually increasing dosage until the recipient can tolerate 100 micrograms of venom, which is considered to equate to two full stings. The conventional method is to give injections twice weekly in a hospital out-patient department, perhaps taking three months to reach the full dose. In this regimen the starting dose of venom is usually varied according to the sensitivity of the recipient, and there may also be variations between different physicians who have developed their own treatment schedules. Personal experience suggests that in all except the exquisitely hypersensitive it is possible to start treatment with 0.1 microgram (μg) of venom, which is approximately $1/500^{th}$ of a natural sting. Thereafter the dose is increased by 0.1μg increments until 1μg is given. After this the dose is increased by 1μg increments up to 10μg, and following that by 10μg steps until the full dose of 100μg is achieved. After a few of these full doses, given at weekly intervals, it is my usual practice to challenge the patient with a sting from a live bee. I believe this is important because many who have become allergic to stings have also become very apprehensive regarding bees. It allays their fear if it can be demonstrated that the sting of a live bee no longer upsets them. Another cogent reason for challenging with a live sting is to confirm that the treatment has been effective, because very rarely a recipient may tolerate full doses of venom by injection but still react unpleasantly to a fresh sting. This unusual persisting sensitivity is difficult to explain. It is possible to speculate that the freeze-dried commercial venom loses some antigenic potency in preparation, which seems unlikely. It might be suggested that the route of administration is a variable factor which could be an influence since the bee injects its venom **into** the skin, whereas injection from a syringe goes much deeper. Finally, many patients are extremely apprehensive when confronted with a live bee and psychogenic factors cannot be completely discounted. Obviously, until the phenomenon has been fully elucidated, common sense dictates that challenging with live stings must be done with circumspection.

Side effects of treatment are not serious, but it should be emphasized that the majority of patients do experience a little discomfort and disturbance at some stage of treatment. The most frequent complaint is of pain and swelling around the injection site. Mild general symptoms such as flushing of the face, slight chest wheeze and cough, and sneezing may occur, usually when the dose of venom is in the $10\mu g$ to $20\mu g$ range. If these symptoms are anything more than trivial, the dose of venom at the next visit is not increased but continued at the same level until it no longer causes any disturbance. After that, the schedule of increasing dosage is continued.

When the full dosage of $100\mu g$ has been attained the conventional advice is that this dosage should be continued at monthly intervals as maintenance therapy for at least two years. In treating beekeepers I have modified this advice by suggesting that as an alternative to maintenance injections they can contrive to get themselves stung every week or two. This may be difficult during the winter, in which case they can revert to monthly injections.

Because the conventional method of hyposensitization is slow some workers have experimented with quicker regimens. In one 'Rush' method which I have used with satisfactory results, the patient is given increasing doses of venom every 15 to 60 minutes throughout the day whilst under careful supervision in hospital. The objective is to achieve a maximum single dose of $200\mu g$ of venom in a few days. Although this can be attained in the majority of patients, the high incidence of side effects has caused the method to lose favour. The considerable cost of in-patient hospital treatment is also a major disadvantage.

After describing so many unpleasant complications of stings it is gratifying to end on a note of optimism and encouragement for those who develop hypersensitivity to venom. In the past, traditional medical advice to beekeepers who suffered serious reactions from stings was that they should give up their bees. Undoubtedly, this advice often caused disappointment and sometimes financial loss. Today, with greater understanding of allergic mechanisms, and convincing evidence that modern immunotherapy is effective, medical opinion is changing. Hopefully, beekeepers with allergy problems will henceforth be given the option of treatment and not simply advised to abandon the craft.

References

1. Abrishami,M.A.; Boyd, G.K.; Settipane,G.A. (1971) Prevalence of bee sting allergy in 2,010 girl scouts. *Acta allerg. 26: 117-120*
2. Arthus, M.N. (1903) Injections répétées de serum de cheval chez lapin. *C.r. Seanc. Soc. Biol. 55; 817-820*
3. British Medical Journal (1981a) Drugs for asthma: mast cell stabilizers. *Br.med.J. 1:587-588*
4. British Medical Journal (1981b) Treatment of anaphylactic shock. *Br.med.J. 1:1011-1012*
5. Chafee, F.H. (1970) The prevalence of bee sting allergy in an allergic population. *Acta allerg.25(4):292-293*
6. Gauldie,J; Hanson,J.M.; Rumjanek,F.D.; Shipolini,R.A.; Vernon,C.A. (1976) The peptide components of bee venom. *Eur.J. Biochem. 61(2):369-376*
7. Gell,P.G.H.; Coombs, R.R.A.; Lachmann,P.J. (1975) Clinical aspects of immunology. *Oxford: Blackwell Scientific Publications Ltd*
8. Hoffman, D.R. (1977) Allergens in bee venom. III Identification of allergen B of bee venom as an acid phosphatase. *J. Allergy clin.Immun. 59(5):364-366*
9. Hoffman,D.R. (1978) Honey bee venom allergy: immunological studies of systemic and large local reactions. *Ann. Allergy 41(5): 278-282*
10. Hoffman,D.R.; Cummins,L.H.; Kozak, P.P.; Gillman,S.A. (1978) Diagnosis of honey bee venom allergy. *Ann. Allergy 40(5): 311-313*
11. Hoffmann,D.R.; Shipman,W.H. (1976) Allergens in bee venom. I. Separation and identification of the major allergens. *J.Allergy clin. Immun. 58(5):551-562*
12. Hoffman,D.R.;Shipman,W.H.;Babin,D.(1977) Allergens in bee venom. II. Two new high molecular weight allergenic specificities. *J.Allergy clin Immun. 59(2): 147-153*

13. Hunt,K.J.;Sabotka,A.K.;Valentine,M.D.;Amodio,F.J.;Benton,A.W.;Lichtenstein,L. M. (1978) A controlled trial of immunotherapy in insect hypersensitivity. *New Engl.J.Med. 4:257-261*

14. Hunt,K.J.;Sobotka,A.K.;Valentine,M.D.;Yunginger,J.W.; Lichtenstein, L.M. (1978) Sensitization following Hymenoptera whole body extract therapy. *J.Allergy clin.Immun. 61(1):48-53*

15. Hunt,K.J.;Valentine,M.D.;Sobotka,A.K.;Lichtenstein,L.M. (1976)Diagnosis of allergy to stinging insects by skin testing with Hymenoptera venoms. *Ann.int.Med. 85(1):56-59*

16. King,T.P.;Sobotka,A.K.;Kochoumain,I; Lichtenstein,L.M. (1976) Allergens of honey bee venom. *Archs.Biochem.Biophysics 172(2):661-671*

17. Lessof,M.H.;Sobotka,A.K.;Lichtenstein,L.M. (1977) Protection against anaphylaxis in Hymenoptera-sensitive patients by passive immunization. Monogr.Allergy 12:253-256

18. Lichtenstein,L.M. (1975)Anaphylactic reactions to insect stings: a new approach. *Hospital Practice 10(3):67-74*

19. Light,W.C.;Reisman,R.E.;Shimizu,M.;Arbesman,C.E. (1977) Clinical application of measurements of serum levels of bee venom specific IgE and IgG. *J.Allergy clin.Immun. 59(3):247-253*

20. Light,W.C. (1977) Unusual reactions following insect stings. Clinical features and immunologic analysis. *J.Allergy clin.Immun. 59(5): 391-397*

21. Loveless,M.H.;Fackler,W.R. (1956) Wasp venom allergy and immunity.*Ann.Allergy 14:347*

22. Lyell,A. (1981) Photosensitivity to medicaments. *Prescrib.J. 21(2): 172-177*

23. Miyachi,S;Lessof,M.H.;Kemeny,D.M.;Green,L.A. (1979) Comparison of atopic background between allergic and non-allergic beekeepers. *Int.Archs.Allergy appl. Immun. 58:160-166*

24. Muller,U.;Johansson,S.G.O.;Street,C. (1978) Hymenoptera sting hypersensitivity:IgE,IgG and haemagglutinating antibodies to be venom constituents in relation to exposure and clinical reaction to bee stings. *Clin.Allergy 8(3):267-272*

25. Muller,U.; Spiess,J.;Roth,A. (1977) Serological investigations in Hymenoptera sting allergy:IgE and haemagglutinating antibodies against bee venom in patients with bee sting allergy; bee keepers and non-allergic blood donors. *Clin.Allergy 7(2): 147-154*

26. Muller,U.;Thurnheer,U.;Patrizzi,R.;Spiess,J.;Hoigne,R (1979) Immunotherapy in bee sting hypersensitivity: bee venom vs whole body extract. *Allergy 34(6):369-378*

27. Munjel,D.;Elliott,W.B. (1971) Studies of antigenic fractions in honeybee (Apis mellifera) venom. *Toxicon.9(3):229-236*

28. Noon,L. (1911) Prophylactic inoculation against hay fever. *Lancet 1:1572-1573*
29. Reid,H.A. (1976) Adder bites in Britain. *Br.med.J. 2:153-156*
30. Parrish,H.M. (1963) Analysis of 460 fatalities from venomous animals in the United States. *Amer.J.med. Sci. 245:129-141*
31. Paull,B.R.; Yunginger,J.W.; Gleich,G.J. (1977) Melittin: an allergenof honeybee venom. *J.Allergy clin.Immun. 59(4):334-338*
32. Pirquet,C von (1906) Allergie. *Munch.med.Wschr. 53: 1457-1458*
33. Portier,P; Richet,C.R. (1902) De l'action anaphylactique de certain venins. *C.r. Seanc.Soc. Biol. 54: 170-172*
34. Settipane,G.A.;Boyd,G.K. (1970) Prevalence of bee sting allergy in 4,992 boy scouts. *Acta allerg. 25(4): 286-291*
35. Solley,G.O.; Gleich,G.J.;Jordan,R.E.;Schroeter,A.L. (1976) The late phase of the immediate wheal and flare skin reaction. Its dependence upon IgE antibodies. *J.clin.Invest. 58:408-420*
36. Thompson,R.A. (1978) The practice of clinical immunology. *London. Arnold*
37. Tiselius,A; Kabat,E.A. (1939) An electrophoretic study of immune sera and purified antibody preparations. *J.exp.Med. 69:119-131*
38. Umemoto,L; Poothullil,J.;Dolovich,J.;Hargreave,F.E. (1976) Factors which influence late cutaneous allergic responses. *J.Allergy clin. Immun. 58(1):60-68*
39. Vane,J.R. (1971) Inhibition of prostaglandin synthesis as a mechanism of action for aspirin-like drugs. *Nature, New Biology 231:232-235*
40. Yunginger,M.D.; Paull,B.R.; Jones,R.T.; Santrach,B.S.; Saritrach,P.J. (1979) Rush venom immunotherapy program for honeybee sting sensitivity. *J.Allergy clin.Immun. 63(5):340-347*
41. Zelenick, L. et al. (1977) Diagnosis of Hymenoptera hypersensitivity by skin testing with Hymenoptera venoms. *J.Allergy clin. Immun. 59(1):2-9*

Facts to remember

- Concepts of allergy and anaphylaxis were formulated a century ago.

- Hypersensitivity to bee venom results from the presence of specific IgE antibodies fixed to mast cells and basophils.

- Immunity to bee venom results from the presence of specific IgG antibodies circulating in the blood and tissue fluids.

- Hypersensitivity to bee venom presents as large local reactions, systemic reactions and anaphylaxis.

- Adrenaline by injection is the imperative treatment for systemic reactions and anaphylaxis.

The following chapter is based on a lecture given at the Devon Beekeepers'/IBRA
Meeting at Seale-Hayne Agricultural College in 1988 and was subsequently
published in Bee World, a journal of the International Bee Research Association,
18 North Road, Cardiff, CF1 3DY, UK

Chapter 3.

Bee Venom Hypersensitivity Update

Although there has been no fundamental advance in our understanding of bee venom hypersensitivity and its treatment since my last review of the subject in *Bee World* seven years ago there has, nevertheless, been some progress which merits attention. Thankfully, for the majority of the population insect stings are nothing more than an unwanted painful experience, but sadly for a few they remain a major hazard causing serious illness and sometimes death. The true frequency of stings and their complications is not well documented but an unpublished Gallup Survey in the UK in 1981, commissioned for market research purposes, suggested that annually up to 10% of the population suffered insect stings and of these 40,000 had symptoms severe enough to warrant further investigation. Statistical information on deaths attributed to stings is available from official sources and average four or five per year in England and Wales and between forty and fifty in the USA. These figures are not necessarily correct; some researchers believe they are an understatement whilst others think they are an exaggeration.

The widely accepted concept of the mechanism of hypersensitivity and anaphylaxis described in the previous chapter will not be repeated here. However, before proceeding further it might be helpful to remind the general reader of the essential components of an acute allergic reaction, classified as Type 1 by Gell and Coombs, especially as it has been suggested recently that the reaction may be adversely altered in individuals taking widely prescribed medication.

Very briefly, the basic pathogenesis of a Type 1 reaction is as follows. Immunoglobulin E (IgE) antibody is produced in those who have a genetic predisposition to generate it in response to certain environmental stimuli. In humans it is produced most readily during the first three decades of life. The antibody is produced by B lymphocytes and is distributed around the body in the blood stream, some becoming fixed to the surface of blood basophils and the remainder diffusing through the tissues to become fixed to the surface of mast cells. The basophils and mast cells are thereby primed to react against the antigen to which the IgE is specifically directed. Exposure to the specific allergen results in bridging of IgE molecules on the surface of the mast cells and basophils which induces changes in the cell wall, activating intracellular enzyme systems culminating in the release of potent pharmacologically active mediators of acute hypersensitivity.

The mediators liberated may have been pre-formed (i.e. present in cytoplasmic granules ready for release) or newly generated following the triggering stimulus. Pre-formed mediators include histamine, lysosomol enzymes and proteases, neutrophil chemotactic factors and heparin. Newly generated mediators originate from arachidonic acid of the cell wall via the cyclo-oxygenase and lipoxygenase pathways and include prostaglandins, thromboxanes, leukotrienes, and platelet activating factor. All of these substances are potent and contribute to the variable features of acute hypersensitivity and anaphylaxis. Some leukotrienes have the greatest bronchial constricting activity of any known naturally occurring substances, perhaps a thousand times greater than histamine on a molar basis. Diagrams illustrating the release of mediators from mast cells were included in the previous chapter.

The origins of mediators of hypersensitivity have been described in a little detail because their understanding makes it possible to offer an explanation for the experience of a beekeeper who reported that when taking Voltarol 50 tablets (diclofenac sodium), a non-steroidal anti-inflammatory drug (NSAID) used for the treatment of arthritis, she suffered anaphylaxis following a sting and blamed the drug for the development of her allergy. Another person reported that she suffered anaphylaxis when stung by a wasp whilst taking Brufen (ibuprofen) whereas previously she had been only mildly sensitive.

Unfortunately, both reports are so inadequate that it would be dangerous to draw any conclusions. It is particularly unsatisfactory that in both cases considerable significance was attached to the fact that when stung again within 48 hours of the anaphylactic episodes, and having ceased taking the drugs, both patients suffered only mild symptoms. It is understandable that in these circumstances the patients should blame the drugs they were taking but it is surprising that their medical advisors did not point out to them that after anaphylaxis there is a refractory period, sometimes described as a state of anergy, which may last several days and during which time there will be little or no response to challenge with the allergen which caused the original illness. Why this important facet of immunology was ignored is not clear but inevitably it brings into question the claim that stopping the drugs was the reason for the subsequent diminished response.

However, despite the shortcomings of the reports, it is important to consider whether there could be any possibility that an increase of sensitivity occurs whilst taking NSAID's since they are so widely prescribed and include the common non-prescription medicaments aspirin and paracetamol.

It has been clearly established that the main pharmacological activity of the NSAID group of drugs is to block the cyclo-oxygenase pathway through which arachidonic acid is converted into prostaglandins and thromoxanes. The lipoxygenase pathway is not inhibited and, therefore, it could be argued that arachidonic acid metabolism is shifted more towards the production of leukotrienes which have great biological activity. (See diagram) Although such effect might change the manifestation of an allergic response, it is not logical to blame NSAID's for the development of hypersensitivity because they have no influence on the production of specific IgE, which is the essential prerequisite for a Type 1 hypersensitivity reaction. All that NSAID's can do is alter the mix of mediators released when an allergic reaction is triggered: they do not cause the release.

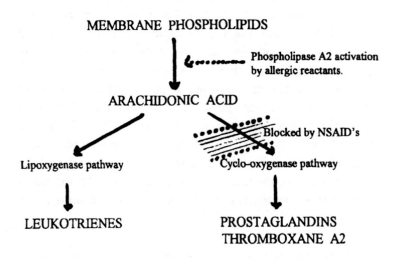

Fig. 1.   Derivation of active pharmacological agents from membrane phospholipids and the site of action of NSAID's.

The above is one theoretical explanation of a mechanism by which NSAID's could enhance allergic reactions. It is not the only one because there is some experimental evidence that these drugs may have some ability to increase mast cell activity. In this context it has been demonstrated that diclofenac augmented allergic and non-allergic histamine release from human leukocytes and rat mast cells under certain conditions *in vitro*. All that it would be prudent to say at this stage is that the interactions of NSAID's with the immune response are still not fully characterized.

Following the initial report asserting that diclofenac sodium caused a beekeeper to become hypersensitive to bee venom, *Bee Craft*, the official journal of the British Beekeepers' Association, .kindly published a letter in which I asked beekeepers who were taking NSAID's regularly to let me know whether they had noticed if their reactions to stings were worse, less, or unchanged. The number of replies was disappointingly small and it would therefore be dangerous to draw any conclusion but, for the record there were 15 replies of which four stated that their reactions were less, two thought they were worse, and nine considered them unchanged.

Treatment

The treatment of stings was outlined in earlier chapters. However, it is worth repeating that stings should be scraped out as quickly as possible and if required a simple soothing remedy such as a cold compress or calamine lotion applied. Anti-histamine ointments and creams are best avoided because of the risk of skin sensitization.

Adrenaline remains the most effective treatment for anaphylaxis, given by injection as described in the previous chapter. It must be remembered, however, that beta-blocker drugs which are frequently used in the treatment of hypertension and ischaemic heart disease will greatly diminish the therapeutic benefits of adrenaline and related products. Those who suffer serious allergy problems and take beta-blocker drugs are at increased risk. Although histamine is only one of the mediators concerned in anaphylaxis it may be the most important. Increased blood concentration of histamine has been described during anaphylaxis and appear to correlate well with the severity of symptoms. Anti-histamine drugs are frequently used in combination with adrenaline in emergency treatment of anaphylaxis, but in order to achieve a quick effect they must be given intravenously. If they are given by mouth an effective blood level of the drug is not achieved until one or two hours have elapsed, far too much delay in an emergency situation.

Anti-histamines do have a beneficial effect if taken *before* an allergic reaction is triggered. Mild general symptoms from bee stings can often be averted if the allergic beekeeper takes a tablet a couple of hours before starting work in the apiary. The older anti-histamines tended to make some people drowsy but with the newer preparations this side-effect is not nearly so prominent. Terfenadine (Triludan) 60mg, astemizole (Hismanal) 10mg, or cetirizine (Zirtek) 10mg have little sedative effect. A disturbance of heart rhythm has been reported with terfenadine in certain circumstances and has for that reason gone out of favour. Cetirizine (Zirtek) is a good choice.

Immunotherapy

During the last ten years hyposensitization regimens using pure venom have been used extensively and have given excellent results in providing protection for many who suffer allergic problems caused by Hymenoptera stings. Details of the basic methods were described in the previous chapter. The question which remains unanswered is how long the treatment should be continued. Some advocate a monthly booster injection of 100µg of venom indefinitely, whilst others suggest that three years is sufficient. Assessments of blood IgE and IgG levels have not been found reliable criteria on which to determine the need to continue treatment, except on the very rare occasion when venom specific IgE becomes undetectable as indicated by negative skin and RAST tests.

My own treatment regimen was designed to help beekeepers and gave good results in a small selected series. A total of 25 beekeepers were treated with only two failures. Those selected for treatment gave a clear history of a general reaction following a bee sting and had a definite positive skin test with venom. Starting in January, graduated injections of venom were given two or three times each week (as described in the previous chapter) until a maximum dose of 100µg was tolerated. The objective was to achieve this by the start of the beekeeping season. The injections were then stopped and the beekeeper told to get stung each week until the autumn close of the season. Throughout the following winter a monthly injection of 100µg of venom was given. The next season the beekeeper again contrived to get stung each week. If in this second season stings were well tolerated no further treatment was given. Those who were apprehensive about their tolerance were advised to take an anti-histamine tablet not less than one hour before being stung.

Before embarking on hyposensitization therapy it is important that candidates should not have unreasonably high expectations of the treatment. Some seem to think that after their long ordeal of injections there should be no pain and not the slightest swelling from a sting. It should be explained that stings will always be painful and will probably still cause some local swelling. It must be emphasized that the objective of treatment is to protect them against serious reactions and anaphylaxis.

Although the initial assessment and start of treatment in my series were undertaken in a hospital situation, the majority of the injections of venom were given by family doctors in their surgeries. As far as I am aware there were no problems. Occasionally, adjustments in venom dosage were required because of minor reactions but these difficulties were settled by telephone consultation.

In the UK in 1986, however, the Committee on Safety of Medicines issued an advisory notice which effectively stopped all hyposensitization therapy in general practice. A small number of severe anaphylactic reactions had been reported during treatment with certain preparations, some fatal. There were no deaths from the use of bee or wasp venom. The major risk was for patients suffering from asthma being desensitized to allergens such as house-dust mite and grass pollen. The report agreed that there was convincing evidence of the efficacy of vaccines to protect against anaphylaxis caused by some antibiotics and bee and wasp venom. Very clear advice was given that hyposensitization treatment should only be carried out where full cardio-respiratory resuscitation facilities were available, and that patients should remain under medical observation for at least two hours after an injection. The implication of these recommendations was that the treatment should be given in a fully equipped hospital and not in the surgery of a family doctor. Undoubtedly, with an ever increasing work load falling on the hospital service and constraints on funding it seems inevitable that it will not be easy to get treatment. Very careful and critical selection of candidates for hyposensitization therapy will be required and in this context the guidelines for venom immunotherapy issued by the Committee on Insects, American Academy of Allergy and Immunology are most helpful. In brief, all persons who have suffered a general allergic reaction to insect stings should be skin tested with Hymenoptera venom extracts. Those with a positive test, or positive RAST test, should be offered treatment. Persons who only experience large local reactions do not require venom immunotherapy, nor should those with systemic symptoms and negative skin tests. There is absolutely no justification for skin testing without a clear history which suggests hypersensitivity, and anyone making such request should be firmly discouraged.

Facts to remember

♦ There is no evidence that NSAID's make individuals more sensitive to venom.

♦ Those taking beta blocker drugs are at increased risk if they suffer anaphylaxis because their response to adrenaline will be impaired.

♦ The antihistamine drug cetirizine (Zirtek) is helpful if taken before sustaining stings.

♦ Immunotherapy with pure venom is effective treatment for those hypersensitive to bee and wasp stings

Chapter 4.

Allergy Problems - A Further Update

(1) Immunotherapy

There is general agreement in the medical profession that immunotherapy is indicated for those suffering serious general reactions such as anaphylaxis following bee and wasp stings.

However, the following are **contraindications**
♦ Significant medical or immunological disease
♦ Concurrent treatment with drugs likely to impair treatment of anaphylaxis i.e. β blockers or other adrenergic blocking drugs
♦ Insufficient motivation to attend regularly and complete the course of treatment
♦ Pregnancy

Treatment is **not** recommended for:
♦ Children under 5 years of age
♦ Those with chronic significant asthma
♦ Those with severe dermatitis

Specific allergen immunotherapy should be administered in hospitals or specialised clinics. Adrenaline should always be immediately available and there should be easy access to full resuscitative facilities with appropriately trained staff. Patients should remain under observation for one hour after each injection.

Adverse reactions to allergen immunotherapy

Injection immunotherapy can induce a variety of local and systemic side effects; these can be immediate, occurring within minutes; or delayed, presenting up to 12 hours after injection.

Reactions to venom usually occur within 45 minutes after an injection. Anaphylaxis is rare and usually starts within 15 to 20 minutes of an injection. Adverse reactions starting after 60 minutes are not life threatening and do not require special treatment.

The commonest side effect is swelling around the site of injection.

Medicines Control Agency - Committee on Safety of Medicines - May 1994 - confirmed that the use of desensitising vaccines in those hypersensitive to bee or wasp venom was effective and acceptable treatment.

(2) Antihistamine tablets

Piriton (chlorpheniramine) is cheap but it can cause excessive sedation. Newer antihistamines have been developed to diminish this sedative effect. Triludan (terfenadine), one of a number of the non-sedating type, was introduced into the UK nearly twenty years ago and has been used extensively worldwide. However, about ten years ago, in spite of a good safety record, there were reports that in certain circumstances, especially when used in combination with some particular drugs, and in patients with significant liver disease, it could cause disturbances of the heart rhythm. It seems likely that the risk of this rare side effect is minimal in healthy subjects who are not on other treatment. However, in the light of current information it is probably prudent for beekeepers to use Piriton providing this does not cause excessive sedation. An alternative effective non-sedating antihistamine is Zirtek (cetirizine). The adult dose of the latter is one tablet (10mgm) daily. It has the advantage of being long-acting, but the disadvantage of being more expensive!

(3) Voltarol and stings

The following is based on an article I published in *Bee Craft* in October 1990 and is reproduced here with the kind permission of the Editor of that magazine.

In the July 1985 issue of *Bee Craft* a letter was published containing the alarming suggestion that Voltarol 50 (diclofenac), a commonly used anti-arthritic drug, was responsible for making beekeepers "violently allergic to bee stings". Furthermore, the writer of the letter quoted her orthopaedic surgeon as saying that "any anti-inflammatory drug is likely to cause this allergy".

It would be putting it mildly to say that I was surprised by this assertion because despite studying allergy problems for more than 30 years I had never heard of this side effect of anti-inflammatory drugs, although I was fully aware that some asthmatic patients are made unwell by aspirin. I naturally concluded that it was a simple matter of my personal ignorance which required correction forthwith! My initial inquiry was to the medical department of Geigy Pharmaceuticals who market Voltarol. They advised me that they did not know of any evidence that the drug enhanced sensitivity to venom. I next approached the Department of Pharmacology of Cambridge University where research has been done on non-steroidal anti-inflammatory drugs (N.S.A.I.D.'s) which is the group of drugs to which Voltarol belongs. They had no knowledge of the problem. Finally, I discussed the matter with two senior colleagues, one a Professor of Immunology, of international repute, and the other a Professor of Medicine who has a special interest in allergy. It gave me some personal satisfaction when it soon became apparent that they were just as ignorant of this matter as myself!

In February 1986 the orthopaedic surgeon mentioned in the *Bee Craft* report,published a letter in the *British Medical Journal* giving some details about a patient who developed bee venom sensitivity whilst taking Voltarol, and about another patient who developed sensitivity to wasp venom whilst taking Brufen (ibuprofen). It appears that a beekeeper, presumably the author of the *Bee Craft* letter, who had been immune to stings for six years, was put on Voltarol for treatment of arthritis. Some months later she was stung on the wrists whilst attending her bees and developed a serious general allergic reaction. The following day she did not take her drugs and again sustained several stings. (It surprises me that she went back to her bees so soon after what was said to be a serious reaction. I would have thought that most people would have avoided them for a while!). Apparently, she had a further reaction but milder than the previous day. Remarkably, she again attended her bees the next day and sustained further stings but with no reaction on that occasion.

Perhaps in passing, I would comment that I find it hard to understand why this lady kept such aggressive bees. What is the pleasure of being stung?

However, returning to the allergy problem, the report is open to serious criticism because it ignores some generally accepted immunological concepts. First, it is well known that sensitivity can develop unexpectedly after long periods of apparent immunity to a provoking agent. In the circumstances of the beekeeper above it could have been purely coincidental that she was taking Voltarol.

The most serious criticism must, however, be directed at the assumption that it was because she stopped taking Voltarol that her reactions to stings 24 and 48 hours later were much less. It is well known to allergists that after a serious general reaction to an allergen there is a period of time following that reaction in which the individual will not respond if challenged again with the offending allergen. This period of time has been termed the "refractory period" and can last several days. In the case of our lady beekeeper it would, therefore, have been preferable if she had assessed her response to stings two or three weeks after her allergic reaction rather than at 24 and 48 hours. Even then, assuming she had no reaction it would still not be acceptable, without further investigation, to blame Voltarol for her troubles, because just as some individuals can become unexpectedly sensitive to venom, others, for no obvious reason, can surprisingly become immune. Allergy is clearly a difficult subject and because our knowledge of it is undoubtedly incomplete it is foolish to jump to conclusions, especially if these are based on a single case. However, we should keep an open mind to unconventional ideas and claims. From that premise, in May 1986 the Committee of Safety of Medicines circulated doctors asking to be informed of any incident where it was suspected that an allergic reaction to insect stings was enhanced by NSAID's.

Because this official inquiry was to thousands of doctors and likely to take some time, I thought it might be useful to make a different approach and ask beekeepers who were taking NSAID's to report if they noticed any change in their response to stings. My request to beekeepers for such information was published in *Bee Craft* in June 1986. The number of replies was small and it would, therefore, be dangerous to draw any conclusions, but for the record, there were 15 replies of which four stated that their reactions were less, two thought they were worse, and nine considered they were unchanged.

In May 1990 I was able to get from the Committee on Safety of Medicines, Department of Health, the results of their request made to doctors in 1986. In the four year period there were 167 reported incidents of allergic reactions to the drugs Voltarol and Brufen (Voltarol 85, Brufen 82). It must be noted that **these reactions were to the drugs themselves** and nothing whatever to do with insect stings. Only two reports mentioned insect stings. One patient on Voltarol developed a general reaction after repeated bee stings. There was no mention of any previous reaction. The other report was of a reaction after wasp stings in a patient on Voltarol. Apparently, before taking Voltarol wasp stings had not caused that person any serious disturbance.

The view of the Committee was that **no** significant problem relating to insect venom sensitivity in patients taking Brufen or Voltarol had been demonstrated.

Addendum

On 2 December 1996 I received more information from the Medicines Control Agency of the Department of Health. I was advised that they had not received any further reports suggesting increased sensitivity to stings in patients taking NSAID's.

After surveillance over a period of ten years with negative result, I think beekeepers should forget alarmist reports about the interaction of NSAID's and stings.

(4) First Aid Treatment by Lay Persons

Many times I have been asked whether a First Aid Box at an association apiary should include a syringe of adrenaline (i.e. Epi-Pen) for use in an anaphylactic emergency. I have always rejected this idea for the following reasons.

Adrenaline is a 'Prescription Only Medicine' which a doctor prescribes for a specified individual patient. It would not be ethical practice for a doctor to give a prescription for a potent drug to be used on someone he did not know. Both from an ethical and legal perspective, the person who signs a prescription accepts responsibility for the appropriateness of that medication. For that very clear reason it is not feasible to expect a doctor to issue a prescription to be used by any untrained lay individual, unknown to him, on unidentified persons also unknown to him.

Anyone who has significant allergy to bee stings would be well advised to seek adrenaline for use on themselves from their general practitioner.

(The above opinion was endorsed by the Ethical Committee of the British Medical Association in a letter to me dated 2nd June 1998.)

It cannot be emphasized too strongly that anaphylaxis is a critical medical emergency for which professional help is required urgently.

(5) Sensitivity to inhaled hive dust

The temperature inside a hive is normally higher than the ambient environment. Therefore, when a beekeeper opens a hive from above, warm air rises from the brood nest into his face carrying with it numerous tiny invisible particles of dust, much of which is organic matter derived from bees, larval debris, pollen etc. This is highly potent allergenic material, which when regularly inhaled by a susceptible beekeeper causes allergic symptoms similar to hay fever, namely, sneezing, itchy eyes, running nose etc.

Like classical hay fever the pathogenesis is IgE based. The treatment of those afflicted is to take an antihistamine tablet well before attending their bees.

Long term inhalation of animal and vegetable dusts are well recognized as causes of serious lung disease in some individuals i.e. Extrinsic Allergic Alveolitis. To date, I am not aware that this condition has ever been attributed to hive dust.

Facts to remember

♦ Immunotherapy is not recommended for children under five years of age or for anyone with chronic asthma or severe skin disease.

♦ Immunotherapy should be administered at a hospital.

♦ The Medicines Control Agency in 1994 confirmed that desensitising treatment for those hypersensitive to bee or wasp venom was effective and appropriate.

♦ There is no evidence that NSAID's enhance venom sensitivity.

♦ Those significantly sensitive to bee venom should ask their family doctor to prescribe adrenaline (i.e. EpiPen) for emergency use on themselves.

♦ Hay fever type symptoms can arise from the inhalation of hive dust.

Chapter 5.

Honey

Honey is the unfermented, sweet substance produced by honey bees from the nectar of blossoms or from secretions of or on living parts of plants, which they collect, transform and combine with specific substances, and store in honey combs.

The major components of honey are the monosaccharide sugars glucose and fructose which together constitute more than 70% of the commodity. Up to 21% may be water. The remaining 9% is made up of numerous other items which include disaccharide, trisaccharide and higher sugars, proteins, amino acids, pollen, organic acids, minerals, vitamins, enzymes and many other substances in trace amounts. Wild yeasts are usually present and there may be fungi and algae in small quantity. Spores of the bacterium, Bacillus larvae, which causes American Foul Brood can be transmitted in honey and very rarely the spores of Clostridium botulinum. The latter have caused fatal botulism in infants.

From the earliest times honey has been highly regarded as a nutritious food and as a medicinal substance. Much of the early information was anecdotal but in recent times there have been some more firmly based reports. For convenience honey will be considered under the headings (a) food, and (b) medicinal properties.

(a) Food

The monosaccharide sugars, glucose and fructose, which predominate in honey, can be assimilated from the gut without undergoing further digestive processes and are therefore rapidly available to meet the energy needs of the body. Glucose and fructose are essential basic components in many metabolic processes of the body, especially as sources of energy in muscle activity. For the vast majority of people honey is therefore entirely beneficial, but not for everyone. It is not suitable for those suffering from Diabetes mellitus, a common disorder of carbohydrate metabolism, nor for the very few exceptional individuals born with specific enzyme deficiencies which impairs their metabolism of glucose and fructose. In addition, in recent years it has been agreed that honey should not be fed to babies under one year of age because of the small risk of botulism. (*See below*)

For most consumers, raw honey has the attraction of being a natural nutritious food uncontaminated with chemical preservatives and additives. It also contains many items, including vitamins and minerals, albeit in trace quantities, which can be considered beneficial.

Sadly, honey is sometimes contaminated with substances and organisms which jeopardize its food value. The following are the more important contaminants.

Clostridium botulinum spores

Classical botulism is a serious acute food poisoning. It was first diagnosed in Europe more than 200 years ago. Originally, the disease was associated with the consumption of poorly preserved meat products, especially sausages, which had been contaminated with the causative organism but in more recent times inadequately sterilized canned meat and fish have been involved.

The causative organism is a bacterium, *Clostridium botulinum*, which is widespread in the environment. Its natural habitat is soil, ground water and mud, but has also been found on fresh fruit and vegetables. It thrives in anaerobic conditions and forms tough spores which are difficult to destroy.

The anaerobic situation inside a can of meat or fish provides an ideal environment for the germination of *Clostridia* spores. Should one of these canned products be contaminated and not adequately sterilized, a thriving colony of *Clostridium botulinum* will soon develop and liberate into the food a highly potent neurotoxin which paralyses the nervous system of anyone who eats it.

The essential feature of classical botulism, therefore, is that the illness is caused by ingestion of *preformed exotoxin* and symptoms appear in the victim within a few hours of eating infected food.

Adults, children, and infants, can all suffer from classical botulism if they ingest contaminated food in circumstances as described above.

The disorder known as **Infant Botulism**, although caused by *Clostridium botulinum*, is quite different from the classical disease in its pathogenesis. Infant botulism involves the ingestion of clostridial spores followed by their germination and colonization of the baby's gut. Subsequently, symptoms develop as toxin is produced and liberated into the intestine. It is only in infants aged under 12 months, where the defence mechanisms of the gut are not fully developed, that spores can germinate. The illness is characterised by constipation, listlessness, and general muscular weakness, often described as the 'floppy infant syndrome'. Sometimes the condition is relatively mild but on other occasions it is serious requiring prolonged intensive hospital care and fatalities have been recorded.

Infant botulism was first described in California, U.S.A. in 1976. Since then it has been identified in many other parts of the world including the U.K. By 1997 the total global count of diagnosed cases was approximately 1500, of which nearly two-thirds had occurred in North America. Only five cases had been recorded in the U.K. up to that time.

Early on in California it was established that a number of the sick infants had eaten raw honey before becoming ill. Subsequent investigation revealed that up to 10% of local honey samples in California contained *Cl. botulinum* spores.

Of the five recorded U.K. cases, three had been given honey prior to becoming ill but there was no evidence that the honey involved contained *Cl.botulinum* spores. One of these infants actually contracted the disease in the Yemen and was flown to the UK for treatment and thereby became included in the UK statistics. A small survey of U.K. honey was conducted subsequently when no contamination was discovered.

In light of the American finding that honey could be contaminated with *Cl.botulinum* spores, Heinz Baby Foods issued a leaflet in 1980 advising that raw honey should not be fed to infants under 12 months old. In 1996 the British Honey Importers and Packers Association was advised that in response to public concern a number of major retailers wished to incorporate a warning on their honey labels that the product should not be fed to infants. Despite all the evidence as to the ubiquitous nature of *Clostridium botulinum* spores the Association felt obliged to agree as much of its honey is imported.

In June 2000 the Public Health Laboratory, Colindale, London, confirmed that although the global number of notified cases of Infant

Botulism had increased there have been no further notifications in the UK and the total of known cases here remains five.

I believe we can rightly proclaim the high quality of British honey. The need to include a warning notice on our labels is arguable but as honey is not an essential food for babies it would seem prudent to avoid feeding it to infants under one year old.

Toxic nectar and honey

It has long been reported that fresh honey from Rhododendron ponticum contains andromedotoxin which is poisonous to humans. In ancient history it is recorded that in 400 BC the Greek army of Xenophon in the Middle East was laid low after eating unripe honey from Rhododendron ponticum.

Other plants of the Ericaceae family are also responsible for toxic honey. Abroad a number of sources of toxic nectar have been recorded but these are not a problem for the UK consumer. Furthermore, it is comforting to know that most toxic substances disappear from honey when it is fully ripe.

It is interesting that toxic honey has been reported in New Zealand attributable to *honeydew* derived from the Tutu shrub (*Coriaria arborea*). Apparently a small vine hopper insect (*Scolypopa australis*) can infest the shrub and feed on its sap. The latter contains tutin, a potent poison which does not harm the vine hopper and is excreted by the insect together with sugars, water and other products to form honeydew. This is attractive to bees and is collected and converted into honey. When ingested by humans, such honey has caused serious symptoms of poisoning and some fatalities.

Following identification of the cause of this toxic honey in 1946 the New Zealand Ministry of Agriculture restricted beekeeping in areas where the Tutu shrub is common and as a result honey poisoning has become rare.

Pyrrolizidine alkaloids

Common Ragwort (*Senecio jacobaea*) was designated an injurious weed in the Weeds Act 1959. Its poisonous effects are said to cause greater illness and losses in British cattle than all other plants combined. Under the Act a landowner can be required to prevent the weed spreading and failure to do so renders him liable to prosecution. Perhaps it comes as no surprise to learn that there has never been a prosecution despite the rampant spread of the weed!

The poisonous principles in Ragwort are a number of pyrrolizidine alkaloids which are particularly damaging to the liver. These poisons are found in all parts of the plant but the highest concentration is in the flowers. In the U.S.A. toxic alkaloids have been found in Ragwort honey and are considered a potential health risk. Australian honey is frequently contaminated with these same alkaloids derived from Paterson's Curse (*Echium plantagineum*). As far as I can ascertain from the literature there are no records of serious human illness attributable to Ragwort honey but there are well documented cases of illness and death caused by herbal teas made from Senecio species.

Ragwort has become rampant in the British countryside in the last decade and because it flowers in late summer when there is a dearth of other flowers attractive to foraging bees, there is a possibility of contamination of honey with these toxic alkaloids. The late Sir Francis Avery Jones, a gastro-enterologist of international repute, was concerned that the intake of only small quantities of these potent poisons might cause liver damage if contaminated honey was eaten regularly. After discussion with Sir Francis I wrote to the Chief Medical Officer, Department of Health, expressing our concern. The CMO was interested in the matter because one of his expert advisory committees was at that time considering the possible danger of these alkaloids in certain 'health foods' especially preparations made from comfrey. He also indicated that the Ministry of Agriculture, Fisheries and Food maintained a watching brief on pyrrolizidine contamination of foods but their surveillance work had been focused on the level of such alkaloids in milk. There had been no monitoring of UK honey. After further representations MAFF Food Science Division agreed to do a study on honey.

The results of a small study became available in 1995. Eight of twenty two samples of honey were found to contain Ragwort pollen and of these eight samples six contained pyrrolizidine alkaloids. However, the alkaloid content was so small that it was not considered a health hazard. The comment was made that the honey samples with the highest pyrrolizidine content were dark, waxy, unpalatable and unsuitable for retailing or blending with other honeys.

The report also contained the further interesting comment that 'little is known about the relative toxicities of pyrrolizidine alkaloids and their metabolism in humans'. In the light of that admission it would seem prudent to avoid them.

In terms of practical beekeeping, Ragwort honey should be avoided because its unpalatable taste can contaminate a honey crop and make it unsaleable. A simple precaution, therefore, is to remove honey from hives in Ragwort areas in late July before the weed flowers.

(b) Medicinal Properties

The medicinal uses of honey can be divided into two categories, namely, (1) local, when it is applied to an afflicted external part of the body, and (2) systemic, when it is taken by mouth.

1. Local treatment

Honey has been used as a dressing for injuries and wounds from time immemorial but only in recent years has factual evidence emerged to explain its beneficial activity.

In the last century it was observed that honey had antimicrobial properties. This was attributed to an unknown substance which was given the name 'inhibine'. Some forty years ago this was shown to be hydrogen peroxide, a potent sterilizing agent.

The hypopharyngeal glands of the bee secrete the enzyme glucose oxidase which in the presence of water acts on glucose to produce small quantities of hydrogen peroxide. The latter breaks down fairly quickly to oxygen and water but its presence is maintained in small quantity in dilute unripe honey by a process of continuous production. In fully ripe honey glucose oxidase has little activity but as soon as honey is diluted generation of hydrogen peroxide increases again. It is the release of this potent sterilizing agent which is the basis of the antibacterial activity of honey. Many of the common bacterial pathogens are susceptible and for that reason there are numerous medical reports of honey as a beneficial dressing for wounds and infected skin lesions.

It is not only the antimicrobial property of honey which makes it a useful dressing. Honey is hygroscopic and as such extracts exudates from infected lesions. This in itself is an important aid to healing.

Despite its virtues honey has never been a fashionable wound dressing in the UK but it has been used effectively in many other parts of the world.

2. Systemic treatment

Honey in hot milk, hot lemon juice, or whisky has long been a favourite remedy for colds and coughs. It has a soothing effect, quite apart from being most pleasant to take. It is used extensively in commercial cough mixtures and lozenges.

Claims are made that honey in lemon juice is a useful remedy for the alleviation of hangovers. The theory is that the fructose in honey speeds the oxidation of alcohol in the liver, and the Vitamin C in lemon juice is claimed to help the elimination of cogeners found in aromatic drinks which are believed to play a part in the causation of hangovers.

Honey in milk was often recommended as a symptomatic treatment for dyspepsia and peptic ulcers. In recent years it has been shown that infection of the gut with the organism *Helicobacter pylori* is a common cause of peptic ulceration. This organism is inhibited by honey and for that reason it is suggested that there is now a rational basis for the use of honey in digestive disorders.

Honey has also been recommended for the treatment of bacterial gastroenteritis in infants. However, it is now most unlikely to find much use in this disorder because of the risk of infant botulism.

Honey and Hay Fever

Hay fever is a common seasonal condition which presents with sneezing, congestion of the nose and itchy watering eyes. It is caused by pollen in the atmosphere to which the sufferer has developed sensitivity (allergy). The disorder shows seasonal variations consistent with the differing flowering times of the various plant species. Many trees and shrubs flower and release pollen in early spring whilst grasses release most of their pollen in late June to early July. Weather conditions influence enormously the amount of pollen in the atmosphere and this makes it difficult to compare directly one year with another. Hay fever tends to be most troublesome in older children and young adults; it generally diminishes in severity with advancing years. With variables such as these, very critical analysis over a prolonged period of time in a large group of patients is required before concluding that a treatment is beneficial.

An established effective preventative treatment for those who suffer from hay fever is a course of injections of increasing small doses of pollen extract. This is normally given during the winter months before plants begin to release pollen. The treatment can be time consuming and not entirely free from unpleasant side effects.

It has been known to beekeepers for a long time that many hay fever and pollen asthma sufferers believe that their symptoms are alleviated if they eat honey produced locally. Some contend that the cappings from honeycombs are even better than honey. Advocates argue that honey and cappings derived from local plants will contain pollens which cause their symptoms and by eating honey regularly they will become immune to the disturbing effects of such pollen.

As far as I am aware there is no confirmed scientific evidence in conventional medicine to support this contention relating to honey.

However, there are reports that give support to the concept that pollen taken by mouth can have immunogenic properties. It was reported in the *Journal of Allergy & Clinical Immunology* in 1997 that microencapsulated ragwort pollen given by mouth was effective in controlling the symptoms of ragwort hay fever. There is also a very interesting report of an homoeopathic trial in the UK. In this 144 hay fever sufferers were randomised to receive orally either homoeopathically prepared grass pollen or placebo. There was a significant result in favour of the homoeopathically prepared grass pollen. Although it is unwise to jump to conclusions such observations give support to the hypothesis that small quantities of pollen by mouth can have a beneficial effect.

To date the view of conventional allergists is that the gut has very effective mechanisms which destroy and prevent the absorption of 'foreign' allergenic proteins and for that reason pollen protein does not gain entry to the blood stream where it could have an immunological effect. In support of that opinion it must be remembered that the average omnivorous human devours a multitude of animal and plant proteins with impunity, which if injected, would cause allergic reactions.

However, for my part, in view of the emerging evidence cited above I have the suspicion that eating pollen may well help those suffering from pollen sensitivity. There is much in medicine we do not know and new information is always coming forward. It would seem prudent, therefore, to keep an open mind. If people believe that eating honey helps their hay fever there is no reason to discourage them. There is no evidence that it will do them any harm and if they have faith in the product it may well do them some good.

Facts to remember

♦ Clostridium botulinum spores have been found in honey and have been blamed for causing infant botulism.

♦ Raw honey is not considered an appropriate food for infants under one year old.

♦ Common Ragwort honey can contain toxic alkaloids.

♦ Honey has healing properties when applied to skin infections and wounds.

♦ Eating honey which contains pollen may help sufferers from hay fever.

Chapter 6.

Apitherapy

The term apitherapy is ascribed to the use of bee products for health purposes. The products concerned are honey, pollen, propolis, beeswax, royal jelly and venom.

Honey was the subject of the previous chapter and its beneficial properties will not, therefore, be repeated here.

Pollen
From ancient times pollen collected by bees has been consumed by man for its food value and for its rather nebulous medicinal qualities.

Pollen contains a number of amino acids, minerals, carbohydrates, lipids, a variety of trace elements and vitamins, all of which are essential for the development of bee brood. Together with honey it is a major constituent of the diet of larvae. In proportion to its weight a larva consumes a considerable quantity of pollen and bearing in mind the very rapid growth of larvae it is reasonable to conclude that a diet of honey and pollen is highly nutritious for bees.

How much pollen needs to be devoured to influence human nutrition is not clear. At the present time it seems to me reasonable to regard pollen as a food supplement but, taken in small quantity, its benefits should not be exaggerated.

The role of pollen in honey for the relief of hay fever was considered in the previous chapter.

Propolis

Propolis is the generic name for the resinous substances collected by honeybees from a variety of plant sources, mainly trees. The buds of poplar trees and horse-chestnuts together with exudates found on conifers and other trees are common origins.

Propolis is a most complex mixture of many constituents, the precise proportions being dependent on availability within the particular locality of the colony. The main categories of constituents are amino acids, aliphatic acids and their esters, aromatic acids and their esters, alcohols, aldehydes, chalcones, dihydrochalcones, flavanones, flavones, hydrocarbons, ketones and terpenoids.

Bees use propolis in a thin layer to coat the internal walls of their hive. It is also used to block holes and cracks, strengthen combs and to reduce the size of the hive entrance to keep out adverse weather and make defence easier. It is also used to embalm hive invaders which have been killed but are too large for the bees to remove.

There is no doubt that propolis has antibacterial and antifungal activity and concoctions of it have been applied to wounds and skin lesions from ancient times. There are also numerous modern reports of the benefit of applications to bacterial and fungal infected lesions. Its use in this way is not, therefore, controversial. What are questionable are claims made by alternative medicine enthusiasts that propolis taken by mouth benefits a number of serious medical disorders such as stomach ulcers, mouth infections, colds and other viral infections, arthritis etc. etc. Those who make such claims have not, as far as I am aware, provided sound supporting evidence from properly controlled clinical trials. I believe, therefore, that it is prudent to examine such claims with a measure of scepticism.

It must be remembered that there can be side effects to the use of propolis because it is strongly allergenic and often causes an unpleasant irritating rash on the hands of beekeepers who handle it regularly. It has the propensity to cause the same reaction (contact dermatitis) when applied as an ointment or similar concoction.

Beeswax

Beeswax is used quite extensively in the pharmaceutical industry in ointments, salves and pills etc. It is used as an inert base or binding ingredient and does not itself possess any direct pharmacological activity.

Royal Jelly

To the layman there is something mysterious and miraculous about royal jelly in its ability to cause a larva to which it is fed exclusively to develop into a queen bee with the potential for a long life, whereas other larvae fed on a more frugal diet of honey and pollen develop into workers with a very short life span. The simplistic conclusion is that royal jelly must contain unique substances which promote longevity and vigour.

With that potent selling line it is not surprising that it has found a profitable market. It has also been sold on the claim that as a dietary supplement it can cure a whole variety of disorders.

Royal jelly is about 67% water, 12.5% protein, 11% sugars, 5% fatty acids, together with a broad spectrum of minerals and vitamins. Clearly, this is a highly nutritious food for larvae but there are no well controlled trials which demonstrate benefit for humans.

In the *British Medical Journal* recently, D.A.T Southgate, head of nutrition and food quality research, University of East Anglia, Norwich was posed the question *"Does royal jelly have any unusual nutritional or healing properties?"* He answered as follows: "Royal jelly has some important properties for the nutritional development of the immature bee larva, providing specific nutritional requirements and influencing maturation and the course of development in ways that are only partly understood. Royal jelly contains a group of biological active insect hormones. These are known to influence nucleic acid metabolism and are essential for the development of the queen bee. The jelly is also a rich source of vitamins. These special properties for the bee larva have led several people to claim that they are operational and valuable for humans. There is virtually no evidence or reason to suppose that the components have specific and desirable properties for man. Furthermore, the amount of royal jelly in most preparations is such that the dose recommended is too low to make an appreciable nutritional contribution to a human."

That seems to me a well balanced and reasonable opinion with which I concur.

Bee venom.

From the very earliest times there have been anecdotal reports that bee stings benefit certain medical disorders. Hippocrates (c.460-359 BC) referred to treatment with bee stings in his medical writings, and Charlemagne (747-814 AD),the military and political colossus of the Dark Ages, is reputed to have had bee stings for the treatment of arthritis.

Surprisingly, with such a long record of use, there is still little firm evidence to support claims for the efficacy of bee stings in human disorders. Although some animal experiments have demonstrated that bee venom has anti-inflammatory effects in artificially induced arthritis in small laboratory animals, there is difficulty in extrapolating such findings to human use because the dose of venom required to produce a similar effect in the much larger human would have to b proportionately increased and, therefore, likely to be toxic.

It is interesting that in this 21st century, which we think of as scientific era, anecdotal reports of the benefits of bee stings still attract coverage in the news media. Scepticism is apparently not new worthy since little interest is aroused when it is pointed out that som well known large-scale beekeepers, who were undoubtedly stung thousands of times during their working lives, nevertheless, develope crippling arthritis. Clearly, bee venom did not do them much good but such negative information is quickly disregarded.

As a conventional physician, claims of dramatic improvement i disorders such as multiple sclerosis and rheumatoid arthritis cause m some concern. In their natural history both of these illnesses seldor run a steady downhill course. The usual pattern of progression i typically by a series of relapses and remissions. The intervals betwee these 'ups and downs' can be very long. I have known of correctl diagnosed patients with multiple sclerosis having spontaneou remissions lasting many years. Clearly, if purely by chance a patie received a bee sting just as a natural remission was about to start it more than likely that the sting would, quite erroneously, receive a the credit for the improvement.

The only way to evaluate whether stings have a genuine therapeut benefit in disorders such as multiple sclerosis and rheumatoid arthriti is by careful analysis of the findings in large properly controlle clinical trials over an adequate period of time. To date, as far as I am aware, this has not been done.

Despite the lack of scientific evidence that bee venom benefits incurable diseases such as multiple sclerosis and rheumatoid arthritis, there are undoubtedly a number of sufferers from those diseases who are convinced that it does help, sometimes dramatically. How can such responses be explained? I suppose it is possible that bee venom has unique properties which have yet to be identified but in the current state of knowledge there is no such evidence so other explanations must be considered. The following are suggested:-

(a) **Chance**

As indicated earlier, if by chance stings are administered at the time when the disease was about to go into natural remission then undoubtedly the assumption will be that the stings caused the improvement. In such circumstances it is extremely difficult to know the truth of the matter. The problem can only be resolved by fairly large scale clinical trial over a prolonged period.

(b) **Placebo effect**

If a group of individuals with a common disorder such as simple headaches are prescribed pills which are said to be a new and advanced treatment, but unknown to them contain nothing but inert starch, a surprising number will declare the new 'remedy' most effective. This beneficial response to an inert substance is described as the placebo effect. It is a common problem in the assessment of new medical treatments and for that reason placebo controlled double blind clinical trials have become standard research practice to establish the effectiveness of new drugs.

In a placebo controlled double blind trial, the new drug to be investigated is prepared together with a second visually identical preparation containing an inert substance such as starch. The two batches are packaged separately with an identifying code on each packet. Neither the doctors treating the patients, nor the patients, know who is receiving the active medication. Patients are allocated to one or other of the 'treatment' groups from a random list. The progress and response of the patients is assessed in the usual way and only at the end of the trial is the code broken to reveal which patients received the active drug. Throughout, patients and doctors have been 'blind' as to who was receiving which treatment.

The above is an example of a simple form of double blind trial. There are others which are more complicated and refined but in essence this rather laborious discipline has been evolved to eliminate both doctor and patient bias and the placebo effect.

Clearly, it must be apparent from all this that the placebo effect is a powerful influence which can distort responses to treatment. It should, therefore, be accepted that some individuals will benefit from stings purely by virtue of the placebo effect, especially if their expectations are augmented by folklore or recommendation by strong personalities.

(c) Urtication and Counter irritation

Roman soldiers 2000 years ago used to lash their arthritic knees with bunches of stinging nettles (*Urtica dioica*) creating a reaction in the skin which presumably brought them some relief. This procedure is described as urtication.

In the 19th century it was common medical practice in this country for physicians to inject irritant substances into the skin over a diseased organ such as a joint. By creating blisters and inflammation in the skin it was contended that the underlying disorder would benefit. There is really no evidence to support this assumption.

The above examples are quoted to give some historical background to the action of some practitioners of alternative medicine who recommend the application of stings over arthritic joints. In such treatment it would seem probable that venom is no more than an irritant and any derived benefit is related to the placebo effect, but regard must be given to possible benefit arising through the mechanisms of acupuncture as detailed in the following section.

Perhaps in passing it is fair to comment on the practice of giving courses of stings, sometimes twice weekly for a prolonged period. If such procedure is followed one of two things can happen - either the patient becomes immune to venom with little reaction arising and presumably little benefit, or the patient develops hypersensitivity to venom with possible serious consequences.

(d) Mechanisms possibly related to acupuncture

The practice of acupuncture varies from the complicated and mystical approach to a crude technique of simply placing needles where it hurts. Acupuncture is an ancient system of medicine which has recently become recognized in the West as a useful method of relieving pain. The precise way it works is still debated but one theory which has much support is that the needles stimulate nervous pathways to the brain where endorphins (pain relieving opioid substances) are caused to be released. The resulting analgesia may last many hours.

It does not stretch the imagination too much to suggest that the insertion of a bee sting may produce similar effects as the acupuncture needle and that the benefit is not, therefore, a specific property of venom.

(e) Endocrine stimulation

The human adrenal glands produce something between 25mg and 50mg of cortisol daily as part of the basic hormonal balance of the body. In response to injury or other significant stress the output of cortisol is increased significantly. It is well known that cortisol and other cortisone derivatives are very potent anti-inflammatory agents.

An injection of bee venom into a small laboratory animal could be sufficient insult to cause extra cortisol release with consequent improvement in experimental arthritic changes which had been induced in its joints. However, I doubt whether a few stings to a human with a much larger body mass is sufficient injury to cause enough extra cortisol release to have a clinical effect. I am not, therefore, persuaded that any benefit attributed to bee stings is derived from a mechanism of endocrine stimulation

(f) Stimulation of the immune system

It has been suggested that some of the benefit derived from bee stings is because venom stimulates the immune system. It is clearly true that the immune system is stimulated by venom because it produces anti-bodies against it as outlined in the earlier chapter in which allergic responses were considered. There is no evidence that such specific anti-bodies have any other beneficial effects.

An important consideration for those giving or advising bee sting therapy must be responsibility. The BBKA legal adviser, Lindsey Bryning, giving advice to beekeepers in *Bee Craft*, October 1999, firmly suggested that requests to beekeepers to provide bee sting therapy should be refused because the beekeeper could be laying himself or herself open to legal action if things go wrong.

In summary, her advice was that sting therapy should be administered utilising bee venom only from a reputable source, of a specified strength, monitored and quality-controlled, and administered by the patient's medical practitioner or alternative therapy practitioner, who carry their own indemnity insurance covering the treatment.

Facts to remember

♦ Honey is a natural nutritious food

♦ Honey has anti-microbial properties when applied to wounds etc

♦ The pollen content of honey is probably of benefit to hay fever sufferers

♦ Pollen has some limited value as a food supplement

♦ Propolis has anti-microbial and anti-fungal properties when used as an application

♦ There is no evidence that propolis has any systemic action when taken by mouth

♦ Royal jelly is of no benefit to humans. A waste of money!

♦ There is no convincing evidence that bee venom has any special beneficial properties in humans. Any observed benefits are probably due to the placebo effect or the mechanisms of acupuncture.

Chapter 7.

Avoiding Trouble

If trouble and difficulties can be avoided so much the better. The following are measures which should help that objective.

The first and most fundamental factor which influences the number of stings you suffer as a beekeeper is the inherent temperament of your bees. Therefore, **ONLY KEEP DOCILE BEES.** There is no evidence that aggressive bees work harder and produce more honey.

If a colony is aggressive cull its queen and replace with a new young queen from a docile strain.

In an urban situation hives should be sited away from public paths and roads so that pedestrians and animals do not cross the flight path of the bees.

In a garden site, face the hive away from paths, preferably behind a 6 feet high screen. Access to the hive should be from the rear.

Open hives in favourable weather. In poor weather when there is no nectar or pollen flow bees are likely to be ill tempered, especially if thunder is about.

In a small garden situation with close neighbour try to open hives when neighbours are not in their gardens. In summer, working in the evening when young children have gone to bed is often appropriate.

82

Always wear a veil. The eyes are too precious to risk.

Keep clothing clean. Bees have an acute sense of smell and are antagonized by sweat and animal odours

Wash beekeeping suits regularly. Apart from accumulated sweat they may be contaminated with dried venom which is likely to provoke the bees.

Do not wear scent or perfume when attending an apiary. They attract bees.

When idly observing a hive of bees do not stand in the flight path.

When opening a hive have all necessary equipment ready and to hand. Work calmly and as quickly as practical. Do not keep a hive open longer than absolutely necessary.

Use smoke judiciously. A smoker should emit cool smoke, not flames! It is not a blow-torch! Colonies vary in their response to smoke, some are subdued with very little whilst others need more. Try to remember any such idiosyncrasy.

If, when opening a colony it seems unusually restless and aggressive, abandon your planned work and shut the hive. Leave it a few days and try again. **Do not fight a colony: work with it.**

Try to avoid getting stung by working calmly and carefully because a single sting will release alarm pheromones which will surely encourage more.

SOME GENERAL POINTS

Only keep the number of colonies appropriate for the site and your own competence to manage.

Beekeeping entails physical work, sometimes heavy. Therefore, choose equipment appropriate to your own physique. Any number of beekeepers suffer from back troubles aggravated by lifting heavy hives.

If possible, mount hives on 18 inch high stands so as to minimize stooping. Keep the back straight when lifting. (Watch Olympic weight lifters on TV- observe how they do it!)

If possible get someone to join you in your beekeeping activities. It makes the work quicker, easier and more enjoyable.

When choosing a site for an out-apiary make sure it can be approached by car. Its an exhausting chore carrying heavy equipment to and from an inaccessible site.

Facts to remember

♦ The single most important fact to remember if you wish to enjoy the craft is **Keep Docile Bees** !

Index

85

Lightning Source UK Ltd.
Milton Keynes UK
UKOW01f1807170915

258792UK00010B/144/P